Praise for

BABY BODY SIGNS

"*Baby Body Signs* is the antidote for the anxiety parents suffer when they notice something unusual about their baby and then worry until their next doctor visit. It is well written and contains a wealth of information not found in other parenting books. It will be an excellent addition to any parent's library."

—JEFFREY L. BROWN, M.D., F.A.A.P., clinical professor of pediatrics, New York Medical College; author of *The Complete Parents' Guide to Telephone Medicine*

"This is one of the most useful baby books my wife and I have come across, and it often cuts right to the chase of what's serious and what's not. As new parents, we find ourselves asking exactly the kinds of questions this book answers. In many situations, unnecessary long hours in doctor's office waiting rooms, long holds to speak to nurse advice call-in lines, misinformation gathered from Internet searches, and serious conditions going undiagnosed could be avoided if all parents had a copy of this book on their shelf."

—NEIL SHULMAN, M.D., associate professor, Emory University School of Medicine; co-author of *Your Body's Red Light Warning Signals*

ALSO BY JOAN LIEBMANN-SMITH, PH.D.,
AND
JACQUELINE NARDI EGAN

*Body Signs: From Warning Signs to False Alarms . . .
How to Be Your Own Diagnostic Detective*

The Unofficial Guide to Getting Pregnant

The Unofficial Guide to Overcoming Infertility

BABY BODY SIGNS

BABY BODY SIGNS

THE HEAD-TO-TOE GUIDE TO YOUR CHILD'S HEALTH,

FROM BIRTH THROUGH THE TODDLER YEARS

JOAN LIEBMANN-SMITH, PH.D.,

AND

JACQUELINE NARDI EGAN

*Foreword by Woodie Kessel, M.D., M.P.H.,
former Assistant U.S. Surgeon General*

BANTAM BOOKS TRADE PAPERBACKS
NEW YORK

2010 Bantam Books Trade Paperback Original

Copyright © 2010 by Joan Liebmann-Smith and Jacqueline Nardi Egan

Illustrations copyright © 2010 by Nenad Jakesevic

Published in the United States by Bantam Books, an imprint of The Random House
Publishing Group, a division of Random House, Inc., New York.

BANTAM BOOKS and the rooster colophon are registered trademarks of
Random House, Inc.

Library of Congress Cataloging-in-Publication Data

Liebmann-Smith, Joan.
Baby body signs : the head-to-toe guide to your child's health,
from birth through the toddler years / by Joan Liebmann-Smith
and Jacqueline Nardi Egan ; foreword by Woodie Kessel.
p. cm.
Includes bibliographical references and index.
ISBN 978-0-553-38565-6
eBook ISBN 978-0-553-90760-5
1. Infants—Health and hygiene—Popular works. 2. Toddlers—Health
and hygiene—Popular works. I. Egan, Jacqueline Nardi. II. Title.
RJ61.L585 2010
613'.0432—dc22   2010001580
618.92

Printed in the United States of America

www.bantamdell.com

2 4 6 8 9 7 5 3 1

To my daughter, Rebecca, who delighted me as a baby and has continued to do so for more than two decades; and to my late mother, Dorothy, who used to say to me, "Just wait till you're a mother!" I'm so glad I took her advice.

Joan Liebmann-Smith

To my daughter, Elizabeth, whose birth made me believe in "love at first sight"; and in memory of my mother, Antoinette Nardi, who taught me that being a mother is the greatest joy.

Jacqueline Nardi Egan

This book is designed to provide helpful and informative material on the subjects addressed. It is not meant to replace consultation with a physician or other licensed healthcare provider, particularly regarding any signs or symptoms that may require diagnosis or treatment. The authors, the publisher, and the *Baby Body Signs* Panel of Medical Experts expressly disclaim responsibility for any adverse effects that may result from the use or application of the information contained in this book.

FOREWORD

One of the mysteries is that as unlike as we are, one human being from another, we also share much in common. Our lives begin the same way, by birth. The love and interdependence of parents and children is universal, and so are the many difficulties parents and children have. . . . Who you are inside is what helps you make and do everything in life.
—Fred Rogers, *The World According to Mister Rogers: Important Things to Remember*

THESE INSIGHTFUL WORDS of wisdom are dedicated by my good friend Mister Rogers to "anyone who has loved you into being." Fred understood well the significance that parents, families, and neighbors have in nurturing healthy growth and development during a child's formative years. Although primarily focused on emotional health, Fred genuinely appreciated the importance of both psychosocial well-being and good physical health. Loving a child into being takes caring, compassion, and comprehension of how to protect a child from harm, prevent disease and disability, and promote his or her emotional, social, mental, and physical health and well-being.

Caring for and nurturing your baby is a wondrous time. Each day brings something new to enjoy. As a parent, you want nothing but the best for your baby. With an understanding and appreciation of certain signs and symptoms your baby might exhibit, you will be better able to ensure good health and a bright future for your child. Most of what you notice is likely to be normal but may seem curious, especially if you are a first-time parent. Some observations, however, may require further investigation and correct interpretation by your pediatrician. By knowing what to look for and working together with your pediatrician, you can make certain that your baby is as healthy as possible and stays that way.

Baby Body Signs by Joan Liebmann-Smith, Ph.D., and Jacqueline Nardi Egan, a wide-ranging compendium of information about your baby—literally from top to bottom—will help you gain valuable knowledge and help sharpen your observation skills. It is presented in an easily understandable manner replete with science-based information and drawings, all focused on providing accurate descriptions of common as well as uncommon signs or symptoms that a baby might exhibit. The authors also present detailed explanations of what these "baby body signs" might signify, all the while encouraging you to see your pediatrician if you are at all concerned.

Baby Body Signs is a wonderful and informative addition to the new family's library. It employs a thoughtful question-and-answer format designed to help you understand which signs are important and what those signs may mean. The book includes clearly labeled warning signs and an important "Signing Off" section that advises you on which signs warrant the immediate professional help of a pediatrician, as *Baby Body Signs* is *not* a self-diagnostic or treatment guide. Remember, when in doubt always check it out with your pediatrician!

Just as traffic signs provide drivers with important information about the road ahead, *Baby Body Signs* helps steer parents toward better understanding of what may be happening inside based on the body signs they see on the outside. With the knowledge gained from *Baby Body Signs,* parents—guided and supported by their pediatrician—will be better able to love their baby into being healthy.

Wishing you and your baby a healthy, happy, and bright future,

Woodie Kessel, M.D., M.P.H.

Dr. Woodie Kessel has been a pediatrician for more than thirty years. He served as an Assistant U.S. Surgeon General and is currently Professor of the Practice of Public Health at the University of Maryland.

CONTENTS

Mismatched Pupils • Misshapen Pupil • Double Pupil • Red Eyelids • Crusty Eyelids • Eyelid Lump or Bump • Droopy Eyes • Double Eyelashes • Baby Shiners • Baby Bags • Protruding Eyes • Too Many Tears • No Tears • Happy Tears • Darting Eyes • Crossed Eyes • An Outward-Drifting Eye • An Up-Cast Eye • Angelic Eyes • Downcast Eyes • Squinting • Blinking and Winking • Lack of Eye Contact

Chapter 4. Your Baby's Ears
Dimpled Ear • Ear Tag • Ear Bumps • Wrinkled Ear • Small Babies and Hearing • Born Deaf • Ear Infections and Hearing Loss • Stuffing Stuff in the Ears • Deafness or Autism?

Chapter 5. Your Baby's Nose
Flaring Nostrils • Hairless Bump on the Nose • Hairy Bump on the Nose • Nasal Crease • Runny Nose • Dangerous Colds • Sun Sneezing • Small Snorers • Breathing Breaks • Wee Whistles • Fast or Slow Breathing • Shoving Stuff up the Nose • Nose Picking

Chapter 6. Your Baby's Mouth
Blue Lips • Baby Blisters • Blackish Tongue • A Groovy Tongue • Heart-Shaped Tongue • Smooth Tongue • Traveling Tongue Patches • Trembling Tongue • Milky Mouth • Crooked Gums • Tiny Gum Dots • Bad Baby Breath • Tiny Teeth • Tardy Teeth • Discolored Teeth • Blue-Tinged Teeth • Yawning a Lot • Drooling a Lot • Stuffing Stuff in the Mouth • Nocturnal Noises • A Raspy Voice • Stammering When Speaking

Chapter 7. Your Baby's Torso and Limbs
Budding Breasts in Baby Girls • Budding Breasts in Baby Boys • One Swollen Breast • Triple Breasts • Leaky Nipples • Triple Nipples • Invisible Nipples • Sunken Chest • Pointy Chest • Belly Button Bulge • Belly Button Stump • Limber Limbs • Bent Thumb • Bowed Legs • Knock-Knee • Pigeon Toes • Duck Walking • Walking on Tippy Toes • Flat Feet • Shuddering Spells • Swaddling

BABY BODY SIGNS

INTRODUCTION

MOST NEW PARENTS—WHETHER FIRST-TIME moms and dads or not—are understandably a bit paranoid about the health of their babies. Babies are tiny, fragile, and helpless beings. If they're not feeling well or are in pain, they can't tell anyone what's bothering them or where it hurts. They are totally dependent on doctors, parents, grandparents, nannies, babysitters, and other caregivers for their well-being.

We all know the classic signs of a sick baby: fever, diarrhea, vomiting, difficulty breathing, and listlessness, among others. But not all babies who have medical problems display such obvious signs. Rather, a baby who doesn't feel well or is in pain may cry, grimace, fuss, act irritable, or refuse to eat. Of course, these behaviors may simply indicate that the baby is overtired, wet, or cold. To complicate matters further, there are myriad medical problems ranging from mild to serious that cause neither pain nor discomfort. A baby may smile, laugh, coo, babble, play, and appear the picture of health, all while there is something medically amiss.

Many medical conditions may, in fact, manifest themselves with subtle signs that a caregiver can easily overlook or deem too insignificant for a doctor's attention. And some of these signs may portend something serious. For example, dark lip freckles can be a totally normal occurrence, or they can be one of the first warning signs of *Peutz-Jeghers syndrome*, a rare, potentially serious genetic condition (see Chapter 8). And while a white forelock may merely mean a baby's been out in the sun too long without a hat, it can be the hallmark of another rare, potentially serious medical condition called *Waardenburg syndrome* (see Chapter 2). On the other hand, signs that look rather scary can be totally benign and nothing at all to worry about. Parents may panic if their baby has yellow stools, thinking that it signals jaundice. But *all* healthy infants have yellowish stools; rather, it's pale ones that can be a warning of jaundice (see Chapter 10).

Pediatricians and other healthcare providers are well versed at detecting both subtle and not-so-subtle signs of illness. When a baby goes in for a checkup, the doctor will look at the baby's head, face, eyes, ears, nose, mouth, torso, and skin, and even inside his or her diaper. The doctor will also ask the parents about the baby's bowel movements and bladder habits, among other things.

But even the most in-depth examinations are likely to take less than an hour. Parents, grandparents, aunts, uncles, nannies, and other caregivers spend much more time with babies than doctors do. So they're often the first to notice something out of the ordinary with a baby—whether it's suspicious bumps on the eyes or ears, excess drool, brittle hair, or some other unusual or unsightly sign. If they pay close attention, these caregivers too can learn how to identify and interpret the signs that may prove serious—transforming their parental paranoia into power. This is where *Baby Body Signs* comes in.

WHAT'S THE DIFFERENCE BETWEEN A BODY *SIGN* AND A *SYMPTOM*?

The terms *signs* and *symptoms* are often used interchangeably. However, medically speaking, a *sign* is objective evidence of a disease or disorder. It is noticeable and describable by others, but not necessarily by the person with the sign. For example, a bulging belly button, which may be a sign of a hernia (see Chapter 7), can easily be spotted by doctors, parents, or anyone else who's looking. A *symptom,* on the other hand, is subjective and can be described only by the person experiencing it. While older children can tell someone about their symptoms—such as a stomachache or blurred vision—babies can't.

HOW CAN YOU DETECT
A BABY'S BODY SIGNS?

Parents and other caregivers can use all of their 5 senses to detect a baby's body signs, which may provide important clues to what—if anything—is medically amiss with the baby.

Baby Body Signs will help you learn how to:

- *Look* for clues in or on a baby's head, eyes, ears, nose, mouth, skin, torso, genitals, and body wastes
- *Listen* to a baby's cries, stomach sounds, and breathing patterns and sounds for signs of problems
- *Touch* a baby to see if he or she has sweaty skin, a fast heartbeat, or a change in weight
- *Sniff* out problems by smelling a baby's breath, pee, and poop
- And even *taste* a baby's skin for telltale signs of certain disorders

WHAT *BABY BODY SIGNS* COVERS

Baby Body Signs focuses on babies from birth through the toddler years, the time when they are still preverbal and can't clearly communicate with others. Divided into 10 chapters, it covers a baby from head to toe, and everything in between. In order of appearance, the chapters address signs related to a baby's:

- Head and neck
- Hair and scalp
- Eyes
- Ears
- Nose
- Mouth, tongue, and teeth
- Torso and limbs
- Skin
- Genitals
- Body wastes

Some signs it covers that may—or may not—mean trouble include:

- Bulging soft spots
- Uncombable hair
- Double pupils
- Sun sneezing
- Triple nipples
- Pigeon toes
- Walking on tippy toes
- Belly button bump
- Blue birthmarks
- Stork bites
- Crooked penis
- Vaginal tags
- Sweet pee
- Green poop

All the medical information in *Baby Body Signs* has been vetted by the *Baby Body Signs* Panel of Medical Experts, which consists of 11 pediatricians and other doctors who specialize in pediatric issues. These doctors are from top medical centers across the United States, and are listed along with their medical affiliations following this introduction.

WHAT *BABY BODY SIGNS* DOES *NOT* COVER

For the most part, we don't address such obvious signs as fever, vomiting, and bleeding. Although we occasionally touch on these signs, they should *always* be brought to a doctor's attention as soon as possible. And conspicuous physical anomalies or congenital problems such as cleft palate and Down syndrome are also not addressed.

We tend not to deal with pain, because when a baby appears to be in pain, it should *always* be brought to a doctor's immediate attention. It can also be difficult to tell if pain is the cause of a baby's crying or distress unless there are other accompanying signs.

Speaking of crying, we don't cover that either. Nor do we address a baby's body language or, for the most part, behavioral and emotional issues. While important, they're outside the scope of this book.

We also don't provide advice on routine child care or health issues such as circumcision, infant feeding, colic, weaning, sleeping, bathing, diapering, or toilet training. These topics are matters of personal preference and/or family, cultural, or religious tradition and are best discussed with the baby's doctor.

Finally, *Baby Body Signs* has nothing to do with "baby sign language," a recent trend in which preverbal babies with normal hearing are taught American Sign Language as an early form of communication.

HOW TO READ *BABY BODY SIGNS*

Baby Body Signs isn't meant to be read cover to cover nor from head to toe. You can pick and choose the body signs that concern or interest you. Each body sign is addressed in question-and-answer format. In addition to the Q&As, the chapters contain 7 different types of useful, interesting, and often entertaining *Signposts*, each easily identified by its own icon. The following are examples of each of these Signposts:

 HEALTHY SIGNS: Signs that are indications of health.

Healthy Sign
An infant's soft spots (fontanelles) should feel firm and very slightly curved inward. When a baby is at rest, you may feel a noticeable pulsation when touching the soft spot on top of his or her head.

 WARNING SIGNS: Signs that may require medical attention and should be mentioned to your doctor. They may also include warnings about certain things that may be dangerous to babies.

Warning Sign
If your baby's tongue changes color—from its normal pink to strawberry red with white spots or to beefy red—it can be the earliest warning sign of scarlet fever.

DANGER SIGNS: Signs that require immediate medical attention.

Danger Sign
If your baby suddenly stops producing tears and has scanty or dark urine, and possibly sunken eyes, he or she may be dangerously dehydrated. Take your baby to the emergency room immediately.

 SPEAKING OF SIGNS: Quotations or sayings related to body signs.

Speaking of Signs
Adam and Eve had many advantages, but the principal one was that they escaped teething.
　　　　　　　　　　　—MARK TWAIN, *Pudd'nhead Wilson*, 1894

 SIGNS OF THE TIMES: Historical anecdotes about the human body and its body signs.

Sign of the Times
In ancient Egypt, teething babies and their mothers ate a cooked mouse to relieve the babies' pain.

 SIGNIFICANT FACTS: Little-known, often weird (and occasionally useful) facts or stats about various body parts or signs.

Significant Facts
A newborn's brain is about 25% the size of an adult's brain and grows very rapidly the first year. By 12 months of age, a baby's brain reaches about 75% of its adult size.

 STOP SIGNS: Strategies for preventing certain signs or medical conditions from occurring or recurring.

Stop Sign
Babies' eyes, especially light-colored eyes, are very sensitive to the sun. But no matter what color eyes your baby has, make

sure he or she wears a hat or sunglasses whenever out in the sun.

SIGNING OFF: This section appears at the end of each chapter. It includes a list of signs that necessitate a call to the doctor or require immediate medical attention. We also include a list of the types of doctors and other medical specialists whom the baby may be referred to for further evaluation or treatment.

Baby Body Signs also contains two important appendices:

- **Multisystem Diseases and Their Signs in Babies:** Some important pediatric disorders can affect different parts of a baby's body at the same time, and are often difficult to diagnose. These conditions and their common signs are described and listed in this appendix.
- *Baby Body Signs* **Resources:** A list of reliable medical resources on the Internet and a bibliography of cultural and historical sources.

WHY WE WROTE THIS BOOK

Our previous book, *Body Signs: From Warning Signs to False Alarms . . . How to Be Your Own Diagnostic Detective,* was recently published in the United States and many other countries. We received a lot of positive feedback from readers who found the book very useful for detecting potential problems not only in themselves but in adult family members as well. We realized, however, that *Body Signs* didn't cover the most vulnerable family members: babies. So we decided to write the sequel (or prequel, to be precise), *Baby Body Signs.*

Babies are not miniature adults, and they often have very different body signs from their older counterparts. And since babies can't communicate with verbal language, their body signs are extremely valuable medical resources; they can tell parents, physicians, and other healthcare providers what the baby can't.

Within a few hours after birth, most newborns are carefully examined by doctors, nurses, or midwives. They will usually be medically evaluated again within a week and then at every subsequent well-baby visit, the timing and frequency of which can vary from doctor to doctor. Unfortunately, there's no national standard for neonatal screening or well-baby exams in the United States. As a result, certain medical conditions may be missed. In addition, some adoptive parents may not have information about what neonatal screening, if any, their babies were given before the adoption. And not all infants are born in hospitals or birthing centers staffed by qualified medical personnel, or at home attended by certified midwives. While Joan's daughter, Rebecca, was born in a teaching hospital with doctors, nurse-midwives, and her husband, Richard (a writer), in attendance, Jacqueline didn't make it to the hospital in time. She gave birth to her daughter, Elizabeth, in her car just off New York's West Side Highway, attended only by her husband, Ed (a businessman)! Luckily, all went well with both babies.

Even when babies are born under optimal circumstances and are carefully examined after birth, not all medical conditions—and their signs—will be present at birth or even show up in infancy. Many baby body signs will make their initial appearance when the baby is with his or her parents rather than the doctor. So it's pretty much up to parents to be the detectors of these sometimes subtle signs.

Our purpose is not to pressure parents into "playing doctor." Nor is it to make them more anxious than ever about their babies' health. Rather, we want to educate parents (and other caregivers) so that they can detect and correctly interpret their babies' body signs. This can help them make rational decisions about which signs require medical attention and which can be safely ignored.

We're also big proponents of prevention; we believe that if there is a potential problem, the earlier it's detected and treated, the better off the baby will be. You can help by paying close attention to your baby's body signs. "Observe, record, tabulate. Use your five senses," said the late Sir William Osler, known as the father of modern medicine. "Learn to see, learn to smell and know that by practice alone can you become experts." *Baby Body Signs* will be your guide.

BABY BODY SIGNS
PANEL OF MEDICAL EXPERTS

KEITH J. BENKOV, M.D.
Chief, Division of Pediatric Gastroenterology
Medical Director, The Children's IBD Center
Mount Sinai Medical Center
New York, New York

WILMA F. BERGFELD, M.D.
Senior Dermatologist and Co-Director Dermatopathology
Departments of Dermatology and Pathology
Cleveland Clinic
Cleveland, Ohio

STEVEN GROSSMAN, D.D.S.
Co-Chief, Pediatric Dentistry
Lenox Hill Hospital
New York, New York

JOSEPH HADDAD, JR., M.D.
Professor and Vice Chairman, Otolaryngology/Head and Neck Surgery
Columbia University College of Physicians & Surgeons
Lawrence Savetsky Chair and Director, Pediatric Otolaryngology
Morgan Stanley Children's Hospital of New York–Presbyterian
New York, New York

BRENDA KOHN, M.D.
Associate Professor, Department of Pediatrics
Division, Pediatric Endocrinology
New York University Medical Center
New York, New York

CHARLES MERKER, M.D.
Director, Pediatric Ophthalmology
St. Luke's–Roosevelt Hospital Center
New York, New York

WALTER J. MOLOFSKY, M.D.
Chief, Pediatric Neurology
Beth Israel Medical Center, New York
Associate Professor, Neurology
Albert Einstein College of Medicine
New York, New York

KAREN ONEL, M.D.
Director, Rheumatology Training Program
University of Chicago/La Rabida Children's Hospital
Associate Professor of Pediatrics
Comer Children's Hospital
University of Chicago
Chicago, Illinois

DAVID R. ROTH, M.D.
Professor of Urology and Pediatrics
Baylor College of Medicine and
Texas Children's Hospital
Houston, Texas

PETER A. SMITH, M.D.
Pediatric Orthopedic Surgeon
Shriners Hospitals for Children, Chicago Hospital
Associate Professor, Department of Orthopaedics
Rush University Medical Center
Chicago, Illinois

CHRISTINE L. WILLIAMS, M.D., M.P.H.
Medical Director, Healthy Directions, Inc.
(Healthy Children Healthy Futures Program)
Former Professor of Clinical Pediatrics and Director of the
Children's Cardiovascular Health Center
Department of Pediatrics and Institute of Human Nutrition
Columbia University College of Physicians & Surgeons
New York, New York

CHAPTER 1

YOUR BABY'S HEAD

Wynken and Blynken are two little eyes
And Nod is a little head
And the wooden shoe
That sailed the skies
Is a wee one's trundle bed.

—Eugene Field,
"Wynken, Blynken, and Nod"

THE TOP OF THE HEAD is usually the first part of a newborn's body to greet his or her parents. Next comes the face, which new parents tend to carefully scrutinize, seeking signs of familiar family traits. But a baby's head looms large not only emotionally but physically as well. Indeed, a normal newborn's head is disproportionately large compared to the rest of his or her body, taking up about ¼ of the body's length.

An infant's head is a remarkable piece of anatomy. The skull of the average baby is made up of 7 separate soft, pliable bones called *head plates*, which fit together like a jigsaw puzzle and are connected by fi-

SIGN OF THE TIMES

During medieval and Renaissance times, babies were both thought of and depicted as miniature adults. Rather than accurately portraying their disproportionately large heads, artists drew, painted, and sculpted babies with an adult's body proportions.

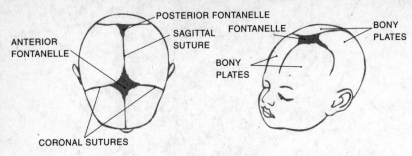

INFANT SKULL ANATOMY

brous membranes called *cranial* or *skull sutures*. There are spaces between the bones where the sutures intersect, which are medically known as *fontanelles* (also spelled *fontanels*), and more commonly called soft spots.

A newborn baby has 6 of these soft spots, located at the top, sides, and back of the head, but only 2 are noticeable—a large diamond-shaped one at the top of the head (*anterior fontanelle*) and a tiny triangular one at the back of the head (*posterior fontanelle*).

Both skull sutures and fontanelles play critical roles during pregnancy and after birth. During pregnancy they expand, allowing the baby's developing skull to grow. They also give the baby's skull the necessary flexibility to make the sometimes treacherous journey headfirst through the mother's narrow birth canal. Then, after the infant is born, they enable the skull to expand to make room for the baby's rapidly growing brain. Finally, the membranes covering the fontanelles protect the vulnerable brain.

Many parents worry needlessly about touching their babies' soft spots because they believe these spots are very delicate and that their babies'

> **SIGNIFICANT FACT**
>
> A baby's heart rate can be determined by observing or feeling the pulsations on the anterior fontanelle on the top of his or her head. These pulsating beats are the result of blood flowing to the brain. Indeed, the word *fontanelle* derives from the Latin and Old French words for "little fountain" or "little spring."

> **SIGNIFICANT FACTS**
>
> A newborn's brain is about 25% the size of an adult's brain and grows very rapidly the first year. By 12 months of age, a baby's brain reaches about 75% of its adult size.

brains are prone to injury. But the membranes covering a baby's fontanelles are, in fact, extremely tough and quite impenetrable. And underneath the soft spots, fluid surrounds and protects the brain.

The size of a baby's soft spots and when they close vary tremendously. On average the one on the back of the head (*posterior*) is smaller—usually less than ¼ inch wide—and it typically closes when the baby is between 1 and 2 months old. The fontanelle on top of the head (*anterior*) is about 1 inch wide, and it tends to close between the ages of 7 and 19 months. Interestingly, this fontanelle sometimes increases in size during the first few months. The fontanelles of boys tend to close before those of girls.

BULGING SOFT SPOTS

Q: Our baby's soft spot on the top of her head sometimes bulges out. Should we worry?

A: It's not unusual for a baby's soft spots to bulge when he or she is lying down, crying, or vomiting; but when the baby is picked up and calmed down, the bulging should disappear. If your baby has a soft spot that *always* bulges, it may be a warning sign of several serious conditions. For example, a bulging soft spot can signal an excess intake of vitamin A. Other signs of vitamin A excess may include drowsiness and vomiting.

A bulging fontanelle can also be a warning sign of increased pressure in the baby's brain from infections such as *meningitis, encephalitis,* or even *Lyme disease.* Or it may signal an endocrine, metabolic, or cardiovascular disorder; a brain tumor; or *hydrocephalus,* which is more commonly called "water on the brain" (see **Large Soft Spots** and **A Large Head,** below). Although a baby with these conditions is likely to have other more serious signs, it's still important to report a bulging soft spot to your baby's doctor as soon as possible.

SUNKEN SOFT SPOTS

Q: *I heard that if your baby's soft spots are sunken, you should bring him to the emergency room. Is that true?*

A: Not always. Sunken fontanelles may be totally normal and nothing to worry about. But they can also be a danger sign of serious dehydration, especially in a baby who has, or recently had, diarrhea and/or vomiting. Other signs of dehydration include sunken eyes, lack of skin elasticity, decreased urine output, and lethargy. Dehydration in a baby is life-threatening and requires emergency treatment.

AN EXTRA SOFT SPOT

Q: *Our infant son seems to have 3 soft spots. Is this normal?*

A: As mentioned earlier, only 2 of a baby's 6 fontanelles are usually apparent. If you notice a 3rd one between the one on top and the one on the back of the head, it may signal *hypothyroidism* (see **Large Soft Spots,** below), which, if untreated, can lead to growth retardation, mental disability, and other serious medical problems. The good news is that hypothyroidism, which used to be a major cause of mental retardation,

---

WARNING SIGN

If you've had an out-of-hospital delivery, make sure that your baby was screened for hypothyroidism. If he or she wasn't screened, have a healthcare professional do the screening test as soon as possible. The signs of hypothyroidism don't always show up until permanent damage has been done to the baby's physical and mental development.

is easily treated when caught early. It's normally detected by the heel-prick blood test that's done routinely just after birth.

A 3rd fontanelle is also sometimes found in infants with *Down syndrome,* but other more noticeable and recognizable facial signs are usually present with this genetic disorder.

LARGE SOFT SPOTS

Q: *The soft spot on the top of my daughter's head is much larger than the spots were on my other kids' heads. What does this mean?*

A: If your baby seems to have a soft spot that looks excessively wide, it may be nothing more than a residual reminder that she was born prematurely, had a low birth weight, or was small for her gestational age. But enlarged fontanelles can also indicate the delayed closure of the skull bones, which may be an early warning sign of a number of serious disorders including *hypothyroidism* (see **An Extra Soft Spot,** above) and *rickets*. Rickets, a bone disease caused by vitamin D and calcium deficiencies, can cause growth retardation, soft bones, and *bowlegs* (see Chapter 7). Both nutritional conditions are medically treatable.

> ### SIGN OF THE TIMES
>
> Although rickets is very common in developing countries, it had been virtually eradicated in the United States—that is, until now. A recent resurgence of rickets in children has been attributed to an increase in the drinking of soy and rice milk, juices, and soft drinks coupled with a decrease in cow's milk consumption. Unlike these other beverages, cow's milk contains both calcium and vitamin D.

Large soft spots can be a warning sign of another bone disease, *osteogenesis imperfecta,* aka *brittle bone disease* (see Chapter 7). This genetic condition often results in multiple bone fractures in babies and small children. Other early signs may include blue or gray *sclera* (whites

> ### WARNING SIGN
>
> Parents of babies that have multiple fractures due to brittle bone disease are sometimes wrongly accused of child abuse. This is another good reason to get an early diagnosis.

of the eyes), discolored teeth, and easy bruising. Although brittle bone disease is not curable, there are effective treatments for it, including medication, physical therapy, and sometimes surgery.

A wide soft spot sometimes signals *hydrocephalus* (see **Bulging Soft Spots,** above, and **A Large Head,** below). Although many babies with this condition also have enlarged heads, it's not always the case. Hydrocephalus can be a very serious condition requiring immediate medical attention.

Large soft spots can also be a sign of several genetic conditions, including Down syndrome and *achondroplasia,* which results in dwarfism as well as other head, facial, and body abnormalities. The signs of these genetic disorders are usually immediately apparent at birth or soon after.

SMALL OR MISSING SOFT SPOTS

Q: *I don't think our baby has any soft spots. Is that possible?*

A: If you can't feel your infant's soft spots, or if they're barely noticeable, it can be a sign that your baby's head plates have fused prematurely. Medically known as *craniosynostosis,* this is a congenital disorder (present at birth). Although its cause is unknown, it's thought to have a genetic component.

A baby with craniosynostosis may also have a misshapen head (see **Misshapen Heads in Older Babies,** below) or a small head, referred to as *microcephaly* (see **A Small Head,** below). Craniosynostosis is potentially a very serious condition: When the skull sutures close prematurely, the brain doesn't have enough room to grow. As a result, the child can suffer from mental and/or developmental deficiencies, as well as eye and other serious disorders. Surgery is usually necessary to correct craniosynostosis.

SIGNIFICANT FACTS

Craniosynostosis occurs in about 1 in 2,000 live births. Males are twice as likely as females to be affected.

SKULL SHAPES AND SIZES

An infant's head has to be very flexible to make room for the baby's rapidly growing brain. But the down side to having a malleable skull is that it can easily become misshapen. Indeed, misshapen heads, or *skull deformations,* as they're medically called, are extremely common in infants, affecting about 1 in 3.

Babies can have any number of unusual head shapes. For example, some babies are born with cone-shaped heads, and others may have skulls that flatten during infancy. The shape and size of a baby's head can be the result of some underlying genetic or other disorder, the birth process, or even environmental or other factors encountered during early infancy. Clearly, babies born with grossly distorted skulls have serious medical problems, but many atypical skull shapes and sizes are much more subtle and may or may not be cause for concern.

SIGNIFICANT FACT

Rather than resulting from a genetic abnormality, about 90% of misshapen skulls are due to external factors encountered during pregnancy, birth, or early infancy. Nearly all of these problems resolve themselves or can be corrected without surgery.

CONE-SHAPED HEAD

Q: My husband and I are very upset because the top of our newborn's head is more pointy than round. What does this mean, and will his head ever look normal?

A: Many parents are dismayed to find that their newborns arrive into the world looking more like a member of the Conehead family, from the old *Saturday Night Live* skit, than a member of their own family. While often upsetting to the new parents, this type of skull deformation—called *molding*—is the most common one found in newborns. Molding is the result of the natural birth process, which forces a baby's head through the cervix and out the vagina. It most frequently occurs in first births; breech births; forceps- and vacuum-assisted births, when there is prolonged labor; and when the mother's uterus is small or otherwise abnormally shaped. The good news is that although your son's head may look weird or scary, it's usually a benign, temporary state. In a few months his skull will likely take on a normal oval shape.

A LONG, NARROW HEAD

Q: *I know many babies are born with cone-shaped heads, but rather than being long from top to bottom, my grandson's skull seems elongated from front to back. Should we be concerned?*

A: If a baby's head looks long and narrow when viewed from the top, it can be a sign of molding *after* birth (see **Cone-Shaped Head,** above), especially if he was born prematurely. A *boat-shaped skull,* as it's sometimes described, is quite common in premature babies. Medically known as *scaphocephaly* (from the

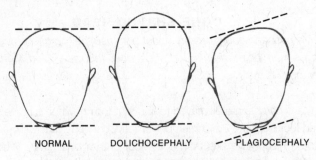

NORMAL   DOLICHOCEPHALY   PLAGIOCEPHALY

NORMAL AND ABNORMALLY SHAPED INFANT HEADS

Greek word for "small sailing vessel" or "rowboat") or *dolichocephaly* (from the Greek word for "long"), it's often due to the recommended practice of placing premature babies on their stomachs (prone) to sleep rather than on their backs (supine). While it's considered dangerous for full-term babies to sleep on their stomachs (see **A Flattened Head,** below), the prone position is the safest for premature infants.

A long, narrow head can also be a warning sign of *craniosynostosis,* the condition in which a baby's skull plates fuse prematurely (see **Small or Missing Soft Spots,** above, and **Misshapen Heads in Older Babies,** below). In this case, surgical treatment is usually necessary.

A FLATTENED HEAD

Q: When we adopted our daughter at birth she had a perfectly shaped head, but now the back of her skull looks flat. What could have caused this and will it permanently affect her looks?

A: A flattened head that develops *after* birth, as in your daughter's case, is extremely common in infants. Medically known as *plagiocephaly* (aka *flat-head syndrome*), it's most often a sign of prolonged external pressure on a baby's head. The baby's face may also have a slightly asymmetric or lopsided look, and you may notice bald spots on the flattened side of the head (see Chapter 2).

While this may sound ominous, it's usually a good sign that a baby is sleeping in the safest position—on his or her back (supine). This type of flattening is medically categorized as *positional molding* or *deformational plagiocephaly*. Although the flattening usually affects only one side of the head, it's sometimes seen on both.

SIGN OF THE TIMES

 Until the 1990s, most babies in the United States had oval or elongated heads. That all changed as a result of the "Back to Sleep" program sponsored by the American Academy of Pediatrics, which encourages parents to place their babies on their backs (supine) rather than on their stomachs (prone) for sleeping to help prevent sudden infant death syndrome (SIDS). The down side of sleeping face up is that there's been an epidemic of flattened heads—a 6-fold increase. Since this program started, though, the incidence of SIDS has decreased an astounding 50%.

A flattened head can also be a telltale sign that a baby is spending too much time playing on his or her back or sitting in the same position in an infant carrier or car seat. In fact, by the time the average infant in the United States is 2 months old, he or she has spent more than 700 hours lying on a firm bed or other hard surface. If the flattening is due to an infant's sleeping or sitting position, it's most likely a benign, temporary condition. While it may be a cosmetic concern, the skull will usually regain its normal shape when the baby is more mobile in a few months.

However, there are some instances when a flattened skull is cause for medical concern. If your baby's head is flattened on one side and he or she also tends to tilt his or her head in that same direction (for example, when held upright or during sleep), it may signal *torticollis* or—as it's more commonly known—*wryneck*. Because babies with this condition usually sleep with their head facing one

STOP SIGN

STOP To help prevent or correct skull flattening:
 • Use pillows or wedges to help reposition your baby's head, but *only do this if an adult will be supervising the baby the entire time.*
• Minimize the time your baby spends in car seats and infant carriers.
• Hold your baby often to take pressure off his or her head.
• Give your baby frequent, but monitored, "tummy time" (prone position).
• If you bottle-feed your baby, make sure to alternate the hand you hold his or her body with during feedings.
• Alternate the way your baby faces when sleeping on his or her back by using visual aids and by having the baby sleep with his or her head at the bottom end of the crib every other night.

side, this favored side of the head flattens. Interestingly, a flattened head can also *cause* wryneck. It's not always easy to tell which comes first, the flattened head or the wryneck.

When a baby's flattened head is related to wryneck or the flattening is extreme, a doctor may recommend physical therapy, or *cranial orthotics*. These skull-molding helmets are most effective when used between the ages of 4 and 12 months. Surgery is rarely, if ever, necessary.

MISSHAPEN HEADS IN OLDER BABIES

Q: I heard that if a baby's head remains misshapen or flattened after 2 months, it can be a bad sign. Is that true?

A: Unfortunately, in many cases this is true. When a baby's head remains abnormally shaped for longer than a few months, it can be a sign of *craniosynostosis,* a potentially serious condition in which the head sutures fuse prematurely (See **Small or Missing Soft Spots,** above). The more sutures involved, the more serious the condition.

When this happens, a baby's growing brain pushes the skull out of shape. The resulting shape depends on which sutures, and how many, fuse too early. As mentioned previously, if the brain doesn't have enough room to grow properly, excess pressure can build up inside the baby's skull, leading to mental and developmental retardation. The

Because a flattened head from positional molding can look a lot like craniosynostosis, it's often misdiagnosed as the latter, much more serious condition. According to the American Academy of Pediatrics (AAP), this has led to a dramatic increase in the number of babies undergoing unnecessary head surgery. The AAP recommends that parents get a second opinion before having their baby undergo head surgery.

pressure can also build up in the eye orbits, causing permanent eye damage. Because of the potentially serious effects of craniosynostosis, surgery is usually necessary.

A LARGE HEAD

Q: *I know babies are supposed to have large heads. But my baby's head seems bigger than other babies' heads. Does this mean there's something wrong with him?*

A: Babies have large heads in proportion to the rest of their bodies—usually ¼ of the length of their bodies. In a healthy baby, the average head circumference is 13 to 14 inches, which is usually about equal to the circumference of the baby's chest. A larger-than-normal head (above the 98th percentile) is referred to as *macrocephaly*. Large heads sometimes run in families, medically known as *familial macrocephaly*. This condition is usually nothing to worry about and doesn't require treatment.

However, an enlarged head may signal *hydrocephalus,* commonly referred to as "water on the brain." This is a potentially serious disorder in which the baby's head becomes enlarged as a result of the leaking of *cerebrospinal fluid* (*CSF*). Hydrocephalus can be the result of a congenital abnormality, a head injury, or a brain infection such as meningitis or encephalitis. Other signs may include eyes that usually gaze downward (see Chapter 3), irritability, excessive sleepiness, vomiting, and a bulging fontanelle (see **Bulging Soft Spots,** above). Although the problem sometimes resolves itself, surgery is often necessary to avoid brain damage or even death.

A SMALL HEAD

Q: Our infant daughter was small at birth and she's still quite tiny. Her head seems small as well. We're concerned that her brain may be affected. Is that likely?

A: If your baby's head is small in relationship to her body, it's probably nothing to worry about. However, if an infant's head is significantly smaller in circumference than his or her chest, it may be a sign of *microcephaly*. In some cases, microcephaly (which is defined as a head circumference below the 3rd percentile) is the result of craniosynostosis, the condition in which the baby's skull bones fuse prematurely (see **Misshapen Heads in Older Babies,** above). When this happens, there isn't enough room for the baby's brain to grow, and surgery is usually needed to correct the problem.

An abnormally small head—either at birth or during infancy—can also be a sign that the baby's brain is not growing at a normal rate. This can happen during pregnancy as a result of a genetic disorder, infections, or other prenatal complications. Microcephaly can also be a sign of *fetal alcohol syndrome*.

When a baby develops microcephaly *during* infancy it can signal severe malnutrition or various genetic abnormalities. Unfortunately, babies with microcephaly often suffer from varying degrees of mental retardation and/or developmental delays.

When these children grow up and have children of their own, their offspring have an increased chance of developing facial or other bodily abnormalities, and may also have seizures. Although there is no cure for this microcephaly, with early detection and treatment many children can be helped to overcome some of their mental and physical problems.

> ### HEALTHY SIGNS
>
> When it comes to a baby's head, size doesn't usually matter. It's the rate at which a baby's head grows that's usually a better measure of health than the actual size. A baby's head circumference should be measured at each well-baby checkup. Between birth and 3 months, a baby's head should grow about 2 cm (just over ¾ inch) a month; from 3 to 6 months, 1 cm (just over ⅓ inch) a month; and from 6 to 12 months, ½ cm (⅕ inch) a month.

HEAD-RELATED BEHAVIOR

HEAD BANGING

Q: *I'm a new nanny for a baby boy who sometimes knocks his head on the side of his playpen. Could there be something wrong with him and is he in danger of hurting himself?*

A: Head banging or rolling can be worrisome, and many people are perplexed by this odd behavior. But like thumb sucking and hair twirling (see Chapter 2), repetitive head movements can be a self-soothing behavior. For example, babies may bang or roll their heads when they are trying to fall asleep. One theory why is that these rhythmic motions may replicate the sensations they experienced in the womb. Like other self-comforting activities, head banging and rolling are quite common and are estimated to occur in as many as 20% of normal babies, usually in the 3rd or 4th month. Boys are about 3 times more likely than girls to bang their heads.

Some babies bang their heads during temper tantrums. It's unclear if this behavior is self-soothing, attention-getting, or both. Head banging and rolling can also be signs of physical discomfort from temporary conditions such as teething or earaches.

Hyperstimulated babies or those who live in an emotionally charged environment may find rhythmic head motions relaxing. On the flip side, babies who are bored, lonely, and lack sensory or environmental stimulation may also bang or roll their heads for comfort. This is especially true of babies who are deaf, blind, or mentally retarded.

Many children with *autism* or *Asperger's syndrome* (which is believed to be a milder form of autism) bang or roll their heads, often for prolonged periods. These children are at high risk of injuring themselves.

In normal children, head banging and rolling episodes typically last for less than 15 minutes, and this behavior doesn't usually cause brain or other physical damage. But some babies who bang their heads, especially during temper tantrums, may inadvertently hurt themselves. And babies who roll their heads may end up with missing patches of hair, some of which can be quite large (see Chapter 2). Most babies outgrow head banging and rolling by the age of 4.

SIGNING OFF

At birth, a baby's head—including its size and shape—is carefully examined by a pediatrician, ob-gyn, midwife, or other healthcare professional. Neurological and other basic functions are also measured by the Apgar test, a baby's first test. Therefore, many head-related conditions can be detected at birth or at neonatal examinations. If, for whatever reason, your newborn wasn't examined at birth, be sure he or she has a comprehensive examination from head to toe by a pediatrician or other qualified healthcare professional.

With regard to head signs, at each well-baby checkup, from birth to 36 months, your baby's head circumference should be measured and the fontanelles and skull shape evaluated. The baby's ability to lift his or her head and move it from side to side will also be assessed.

However, parents may be the first to notice some important, perhaps even life-threatening, head-related or neurological problems.

CALL YOUR BABY'S DOCTOR OR 911 IMMEDIATELY IF YOUR BABY:

- Has a soft spot (or spots) that bulges or sinks suddenly
- Has a convulsion (seizure)
- Has just had a severe blow to the head or other head injury
- Is unresponsive or can't be awakened
- Suddenly can't lift his or her head
- Suddenly becomes uncoordinated
- Seems dizzy or disoriented
- Seems to have sudden severe head pain (especially when accompanied by vomiting and/or a high fever)

SIGN OF THE TIMES

The Apgar test and score were named for Dr. Virginia Apgar, the American physician who devised the test in 1952.

APGAR also stands for American Pediatric Gross Assessment Record.

In addition, the letters spell out the health signs evaluated in a newborn:

- **A**ppearance (skin color)
- **P**ulse (heart rate)
- **G**rimace (reflex irritability)
- **A**ctivity (muscle tone)
- **R**espiration

The letters represent the same things in German, Spanish, and French.

A baby with a neurological or other head-related problem may be referred to a pediatric neurologist or other specialist.

CHAPTER 2

YOUR BABY'S HAIR AND SCALP

There was a little girl,
Who had a little curl,
Right in the middle of her forehead.
When she was good,
She was very good indeed.
But when she was bad,
She was horrid.
—Henry Wadsworth Longfellow,
"There Was a Little Girl"

MANY BABIES ARE BORN BALD, while others come into the world with a few wisps or even a full head of hair. Babies may have a mop of curls or hair as straight as a porcupine's quills. And the texture of their hair may be smooth as silk or coarse as straw. All of this, and we haven't even begun to talk about the wide range of colors babies' hair can have!

A fetus begins to show signs of hair growth as early as the 8th week of pregnancy. By the 10th week, hair follicles on the scalp begin to appear,

SIGN OF THE TIMES

An old wives' tale says women who have heartburn during pregnancy give birth to babies with lots of hair. Recently researchers reported in the medical journal *Birth* that there's truth in the locks lore. Indeed, the more severe the mother's heartburn, the more hair her newborn has.

and by 5 to 6 months, all of the developing hair follicles are formed. In total, out of the 5 million hair follicles on the body, 1 million are on the head and scalp. Remarkably, no further follicles are formed either before or after birth, meaning that most of the scalp hair a baby has at birth is already several months old.

Fetuses are covered with *lanugo,* a downy, light-colored hair that's usually shed before birth in full-term babies. (In fact, the presence of lanugo in a newborn is a sign of a premature birth.) Most full-term newborns are covered with short, fine, silky hair, which has replaced lanugo. These *vellus* hairs, as they're called, cover most of a baby's head and body, with the exception of the palms of the hands, soles of the feet, eyelids, lips, and tip of the penis, to name a few spots. Although the peach-fuzzy vellus hair usually continues to grow, making up one-quarter of a baby's scalp hair, it's usually not noticed because of its light color.

However a baby's hair looks when it first grows in, most parents can't resist clipping a lock as a keepsake. While they might not realize it, that lock of hair can unlock clues to a variety of genetic, nutritional, metabolic, and other medical conditions.

> ### SIGNIFICANT FACT
>
> A baby's cowlick is a left-over sign of brain growth while in the womb. The hair whorl is created when the scalp stretches to accommodate the growing brain. Hair whorls are usually clockwise spirals, and most are on the left side (probably because the left side of the brain is larger than the right).

> ### SIGN OF THE TIMES
>
> A Russian company specializing in producing gem-quality synthetic diamonds advertises that it can turn baby hair into fake diamonds! Pet hair also works well. Like babies (or pets), these little gems are precious and costly too.

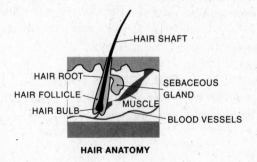

HAIR SHAFT

HAIR ROOT

HAIR FOLLICLE

HAIR BULB

SEBACEOUS GLAND

MUSCLE

BLOOD VESSELS

HAIR ANATOMY

HAIR COLOR

Hair color is largely the result of genetics. But figuring out exactly what color hair your baby will have at birth and as an adult isn't easy, even for geneticists. A baby's hair may be black, brown, blond, or red—or a spectrum of shades in between—depending on his or her racial and ethnic background.

Black is the most common hair color in the world, occurring in people of all races and ethnicities. Brown comes in at a close second, found mostly in those of European, Middle Eastern, African, and Latino heritage. Only about 2% of the world's population has naturally blond hair. Strawberry blond is even rarer and is usually seen in those of British descent. Rarest of all is red hair, which is seen in less than 2% of the world's population.

Like eye and skin color, a baby's hair color depends primarily on how much *melanin* (the color-producing pigment) he or she has inherited. Regardless of what color hair a baby has at birth, it will most likely darken during the first 5 to 10 years of life. Therefore, your adorable little Goldilocks may end up a brown-haired beauty.

SIGN OF THE TIMES

In mid-2007, a rumor spread around the world that redheads would be extinct by the year 2060! This tall tale was based on the misinterpretation of information appearing in *National Geographic*. The original article had merely reiterated the rarity of redheads, not predicted their impending demise.

SIGN OF THE TIMES

In the early 20th century, laypeople and doctors alike thought that children with red hair were susceptible to rheumatic fever. Indeed, the man referred to as the father of English pediatrics, Sir George Frederic Still, reported an unusually large number of redheaded children with rheumatism. Today, that association is no longer considered valid.

COLORLESS HAIR

Q: *My sister and I come from a long line of brunettes, but my newborn niece's hair is so light, it's almost white. Will it darken, or might she be an albino?*

A: Your niece may be one of those natural—but often temporary—platinum blondes who are known as "towheads." True towheads nearly always end up with darker hair, while the hair of children with albinism stays very light throughout life. If your niece were an albino, her eyes and skin would have little or no color as well. (The hair of albinos of African or Asian descent may have a yellow, red, or brown tint instead of being colorless.)

Albinism, which is a defect in the pigment-producing cells (*melanocytes*), is an inherited condition. But just because no one in your family has it doesn't mean that your niece or another child in your family won't inherit it. Most albino children are actually born to parents with normal hair, eye, and skin color. Both parents, however, have to carry one copy of the abnormal gene for their baby to have albinism.

Although albino children are totally healthy, nearly all have abnormal vision, which can range from mild impairment to being legally blind. Albinism can also be associated with other eye problems such as involuntary eye movements, known as *nystagmus,* or eye alignment problems, known as *strabismus*. (See Chapter 3.) And because their skin and eyes are so light, they're at increased risk for sunburn and they usually require special precautions when in the sun.

SIGN OF THE TIMES

The use of the term *towhead* to describe a very light blonde can trace its roots to colonial times. Flax, a pale fiber used to make fabric, was pulled or "combed" through a bed of nails in a process called "towing." The shorter fibers were called "tow," and people, especially children, with short, light-colored hair got nicknamed "towheads."

A WHITE STREAK OF HAIR

Q: Our baby was born with a patch of white hair right in the front of his forehead. It seems unusual. What can cause this, and is it something to worry about?

A: A streak of white hair on a forehead is commonly called a *forelock* and is medically known as *poliosis*. This rather scary-sounding medical term applies to small patches of white hair on the head or any other part of the body. (Fortunately, poliosis has nothing to do with the once-dreaded, contagious viral infection *poliomyelitis,* which can cause paralysis.)

In rare cases, white forelocks may be a sign of the genetic condition *piebaldism,* in which some pigment-producing cells (*melanocytes*) don't develop normally. Some babies with piebaldism may also have a triangular or diamond-shaped patch of chalk-white skin under the forelock and/or colorless hairs in the middle of their eyebrows and eyelashes. Piebaldism, which often runs in families, doesn't usually worsen. In fact, the colorless areas occasionally get smaller with time.

While a white forelock is often benign, it is also one of the classic signs of a rare but potentially serious hereditary condition called *Waardenburg syndrome* (*WS*). Eyebrows that grow together across the bridge of the nose, a condition called *synophrys,* are another hair sign of WS, which can also affect the eyes and skin. (See Chapters 3 and 8.) Hearing loss is also a quite common sign. In the more serious forms of this disorder, babies have other more obvious and serious physical signs such as a cleft palate and other facial deformities.

While there is no specific medical treatment for Waardenburg syndrome, many approaches are available to help manage some of the vision, hearing, and other problems it can cause.

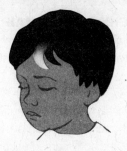

WHITE FORELOCK (POLIOSIS)

HAIR TEXTURE

Like the color of your baby's hair, whether your son or daughter will ultimately end up with curly, wavy, straight, thick, or fine hair is also based on genetics. People of African heritage tend to have tightly curled or spiral hair, whereas Asians usually have coarse, thick, straight hair. The hair of whites is often thinner than that of other races and can be straight, wavy, or curly.

Many parents notice a change in their baby's hair texture at about 3 to 7 months of age, and by the 2nd birthday, a baby's hair is likely to have thickened. If a baby's hair texture is very different from the rest of the family's, styling or other external factors may be to blame. But it may also be a warning sign of a medical problem that the baby was either born with or developed later in life.

SPEAKING OF SIGNS

 It is not to tease you and hurt you, my Sweet,
But only for kindness and care,
That I wash you, and dress you,
and make you look neat,
And comb out your tanglesome hair.

— Anonymous

SIGNS OF THE TIMES

 To ensure that a baby has curly hair:

- During pregnancy, the expectant mother should cut off several of her curls and bury them.
- The baby should be wrapped in fur before being dressed for the first time.
- Every night for a week following birth, a silk handkerchief should be rubbed over the baby's head.

— American old wives' tales

VERY TANGLY HAIR

Q: *For my 18-month-old adopted daughter, every day seems like a bad hair day. I can't even put a comb through her hair. Could something be wrong with her?*

A: Many parents occasionally find it a challenge to untangle their babies' knotted hair. But if your baby's hair is usually an unruly, snarly mass, it may be a sign of the aptly named *uncombable hair syndrome* (*UHS*). Although rare and benign when it stands alone, this syndrome has managed to rack up a myriad of medical monikers, including *spun-glass hair syndrome, cheveux incoiffables,* and *pili trianguli et canaliculi syndrome.* Usually UHS becomes apparent in children 3 to 12 months of age. Although it tends to run in families, not all children with UHS have relatives who've had the same problem.

UHS usually affects all scalp hair, although sometimes only small patches of wiry hair are affected. The frizzy hair, which is typically silvery blond or straw-colored, actually takes on a spun-glass appearance; some of its strands will seem to glisten. Although the hair is usually dry and coarse, it's not fragile. But tugging on it during combing can yank out clumps. Sometimes special hair products may help calm down the wild and crazy hair until the child outgrows this condition—usually at puberty.

Unmanageable hair can also be a sign of another hair shaft disorder called *loose anagen hair syndrome,* a condition in which strands of hair can be pulled out effortlessly. (See **Hair That Pulls Out Easily,** below.) Unbecoming, uncombable hair is primarily a cosmetic issue not associated with any physical or neurological problems. However, in rare cir-

---

WARNING SIGN

Estrogen- or placenta-containing hair and skin products are quite popular, especially among African American women. They should *never* be used on children of any age. Researchers believe that using them during pregnancy and on babies may explain why African American children are at increased risk of premature puberty.

cumstances, UHS is seen in children who have *ectodermal dysplasia syndrome (EDS)*, which is actually a group of more than 150 hereditary disorders that affect the body's tissues. Children with EDS can be born with mild to serious defects in their teeth, skin, nails, and other body parts. While there's no cure, many treatments are available to help alleviate EDS-related problems.

EASILY BROKEN HAIR

Q: My 2-year-old granddaughter's hair seems very fragile and breaks off easily. What could be the problem?

A: A toddler's hair may repeatedly break from a variety of external, environmental, or even emotional events. Some examples include vigorous shampooing (especially with harsh shampoos), overbrushing, blow-drying, head banging or rolling (see Chapter 1 and **Baby Bald Patch,** below), and hair twirling (see **Hair Twirling,** below). And babies with scalp infections, such as *seborrheic dermatitis* (see **White Flakes on the Scalp,** below), may scratch their heads, causing susceptible strands of hair to break off.

All of the factors above, as well as other hair trauma, can be signs of a common fragile hair shaft disorder called *trichorrhexis nodosa*. Depending on the type of hair a child has, trichorrhexis nodosa can affect them differently. For example, in children of African descent and in others with tight curls, the hair tends to break off very close to the scalp, leaving noticeable bald spots. On the other hand, the hair of white or Asian children who have this problem tends to break midstrand or toward the ends.

Babies can also be born with fragile hair. In these cases, the hair breaks with even a tiny bit of tugging. For instance, when hair is both fragile and lackluster it may be an inherited type of trichorrhexis no-dosa known as *bamboo hair* (aka *trichorrhexis invaginata*). Bamboo hair usually shows up in infancy and is more common in girls than boys. Besides being fragile and dull, the hair is usually, dry, flat, short, and sparse. Fortunately, many children with bamboo hair start growing normal hair by the time they enter school. But this condition can persist through puberty, which may adversely affect a child's self-image.

SIGNIFICANT FACT

Bamboo hair is so named because it looks like a stalk of bamboo under a microscope (but not to the naked eye).

SIGNIFICANT FACT

The term *monilethrix* comes from the Latin *monile*, "necklace," and the Greek *thrix*, "hair." Under a microscope the hair looks like a string of beads.

Fragile, dull, and/or brittle hair can also be a sign of another rare inherited disorder called *monilethrix*, which is usually first noticed a few months after birth. With this condition, the baby's growing hair keeps breaking and never reaches more than a few inches. This leaves little hair stubs on the scalp, which may have a burnt appearance.

Monilethrix affects mainly scalp hair and may be worse on the back of the head and nape of the neck. Sometimes the eyelashes, eyebrows, and hair on other parts of the body are affected as well. This hair disorder can also cause some hair loss, and the scalp may be crusty or scaly. While monilethrix never totally goes away, it sometimes improves during puberty.

Regardless of the cause of fragile hair, for the most part it's a benign, cosmetic condition. A little tender loving care will usually straighten out any problem.

WARNING SIGN

Fragile bamboo hair along with thick, flaking skin and red rashes may be signs of *Netherton's syndrome,* a serious inherited condition, which may or may not be apparent at birth. Children with this disorder often have allergies and repeated infections.

HAIR THAT PULLS OUT EASILY

Q: *I'm the new nanny for a 2-year-old girl. When I comb her hair, even very gently, clumps of hair come out. What gives?*

A: There's a recently identified condition called *loose anagen hair syndrome* (*LAHS*), in which hair pulls out easily and painlessly from the scalp. The exact cause of this benign but cosmetically concerning condition is unknown, although it occasionally runs in families. The typical child with LAHS is a 2- to 5-year-old girl with blond hair. It's seen primarily in whites.

When babies with LAHS rub their heads against a pillow or car seat, their hair is likely to become loose and fall out. (See **Baby Bald Patch,** below.) As a result, their hair may not grow very long. In fact, parents often don't suspect anything is amiss until they realize they've rarely, if ever, cut their baby's hair.

Luckily, this hair problem is usually temporary. It will typically improve or disappear altogether by the time the child reaches adolescence.

HAIR THAT ISN'T THERE

As mentioned earlier, it's not uncommon for babies to be born bald. Nor it is unusual for babies to lose much or all of their hair during the first few months of life. In fact, new mothers may notice that their baby's hair loss parallels the very common postpartum hair loss they themselves may be experiencing. Luckily, both Mom's hair and Baby's hair will regrow.

WARNING SIGN

Medical journals have reported rather unusual and sometimes dangerous effects of postpartum hair loss. A loose strand of a new mom's hair can wrap tightly around her baby's toes, causing a condition called *hair-thread tourniquet syndrome.* There have also been reports of hair strands wrapping around a baby's penis, which is a far more perilous situation. Moms with long hair should be particularly cautious about where their shedding postpartum hair lands.

But there are other reasons—some benign, some serious—why babies may be born without hair or lose it after birth, medically referred to as *alopecia*. The pattern of hair loss and whether it occurs with redness, swelling, scaling, or even pus are all signs that can pinpoint the cause of the shedding.

BORN BALD

Q: My grandson was born as bald as a cue ball. He's 9 months old but his hair still hasn't started growing. Isn't that unusual?

A: It's quite unusual for babies to be born without any hair. Most newborns, whether born "bald" or not, actually have some fuzzlike hair (*vellus*) on their heads. This fine, barely noticeable hair is then replaced by thicker and more textured hair, called *terminal hair.* Depending on a baby's genes or other factors, it may take a couple of months, or even a year or more, for this hair to grow in.

In very rare cases, a baby may be born without any vellus hair, a condition medically known as *congenital hypotrichosis,* which is sometimes called *alopecia congenitalis*. If the child never develops body hair, including eyebrows and eyelashes, it's referred to as *alopecia universalis*. (These are misnomers, since *alopecia* refers to hair that was initially present and then lost.)

Congenital hypotrichosis is usually caused by a genetic flaw or a defect that occurs during embryonic development. In some cases, only a portion of the hair is missing. (See **Triangular Bald Spot,** below.) When hypotrichosis affects the whole head, it's usually associated with other more serious and obvious physical deformities and developmental problems. While there may be treatment for some underlying conditions, none is available for hypotrichosis.

WARNING SIGN

While it's perfectly normal for babies to lose their first hair shortly after birth, hair loss after they turn about 6 months of age is not. Be sure to bring it to the attention of your baby's doctor.

TRIANGULAR BALD SPOT

Q: Our toddler has hair all over his head except for an arrow-shaped spot on the side. What could have caused this?

A: It sounds like your son may have a benign, fairly uncommon condition called *congenital temporal triangular alopecia,* which is a form of *congenital hypotrichosis* (see **Born Bald,** above). As the name implies, babies with this condition usually have a triangular patch of hair missing from the temples. That said, the missing patch of hair can be oval, round, or virtually any shape. In rare instances, several patches may be missing from around the temples.

Because many babies don't have much hair anyway, parents may not even notice this problem until their baby is 2 or 3 years old. Although the hair loss is permanent, the good news is that the hairless area or areas won't get any bigger. And as the rest of the child's hair grows in, it can be styled to cover the bald spots.

BABY BALD PATCH

Q: Our 3-month-old has a hunk of hair missing. What could have caused this and will her hair eventually grow?

A: Hair that's missing from the back or side of a baby's head may be a telltale sign of *friction* or *pressure alopecia.* This is a benign condition in which hair falls out because of repeated rubbing against objects such as a playpen mattress or car seat padding. And when babies are put in one position for prolonged periods, it can place pressure on their heads, leading to a paucity of hair. Indeed, if your daughter's hair is missing from the back of her head, it can be a healthy sign that she's sleeping in the safest position for most babies — on her back. The back of her head may also look a bit flattened. (See Chapter 1.)

> ### SIGN OF THE TIMES
>
> Patches of lost hair are becoming quite common among babies as many parents are heeding the recommendations of the recent public-health "Back to Sleep" campaign and are placing their infants to sleep on their backs. This is an important step toward decreasing the risk of *sudden infant death syndrome* (SIDS).

Babies and toddlers who are head bangers (see Chapter 1) can also end up with these types of bald spots. In cases of friction- and pressure-related bald patches, when the rubbing, pressure, or banging stops, the hair will usually grow back.

WARNING SIGN

Excessive brushing, braiding, or twisting, as well as tight barrettes, pigtails, or dreadlocks, can cause a type of hair loss called *traction alopecia*. Fortunately, the hair usually grows back normally when the overly rigorous styling stops.

BALDING BABY

Q: Our toddler is suddenly losing the hair on his head. What could this mean?

A: Your son may have *alopecia areata*, one of the most common causes of hair loss in children, affecting about 1 in 1,000. This type of hair loss, which usually happens rather quickly, rarely occurs in children younger than 18 months. The distinguishing signs of alopecia areata are a totally (or nearly totally) hairless, smooth, round area of skin where hair once was. One or several patches of hair may be missing. The skin in these patches will not be inflamed or scaly. The surrounding area may have stubbles, referred to as *exclamation marks,* which should not be confused with the broken hairs called *black dot sign* seen in babies with ringworm. (See **Spotted, Scaly Scalp,** below.)

Alopecia areata (which also affects adults) is considered an autoimmune condition in which the body's immune system mistakenly attacks its hair follicles. It's thought to be an inherited condition, but it's totally different from *male-pattern baldness,* the type of baldness most common in men, which is also inherited. Alopecia areata tends to run in families with a history of asthma, hay fever, eczema, and childhood diabetes. It's also seen in families with such autoimmune disorders as thyroid disease and *vitiligo,* a condition in which the skin develops white patches (see Chapter 8). Although it's usually just a cosmetic concern, children (and adults) with alopecia areata may be at increased risk for these other genetic and/or autoimmune disorders. And a small percentage of babies with this condition will go on to develop *alopecia totalis,* the total loss of scalp hair, or even *alopecia universalis,* the loss of all body hair (see **Born Bald,** above).

STOP SIGN

 Bald babies and those who have lost large amounts of head hair are at risk for sunburned scalps. They should wear a hat, as well as sunscreen, whenever they're out in the sun.

While there's no cure for alopecia areata, sometimes corticosteroids and other medical ointments are prescribed. But the bald spot, especially if small, may fill in after a few months. In general, the more hair that's lost, the less likely it is that it will grow back. And if it does grow in, it's more likely to fall out again.

WARNING SIGN

 While hair loss can signal a benign or serious medical condition, so can excessive hair (*hypertrichosis*). More-than-normal amounts of hair—or hair in unusual places—can be a telltale sign of a genetic disorder, a hormonal imbalance, a drug reaction, or fetal alcohol syndrome.

Hair loss in a toddler can also signal another, much less common form of alopecia called *telogen effluvium*. In this condition, there's extensive but temporary shedding of head hair. The hair actually comes out from the roots. Telogen effluvium doesn't usually run in families. Rather, it can be caused by a variety of physical or emotional traumas, such as

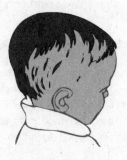

TELOGEN EFFLUVIUM

prolonged high fevers, surgery, serious infections, nutritional deficiencies, or severe stress. The hair usually falls out about 3 months after such events. It can also be a reaction to a drug, radiation, or chemotherapy. This is the same type of hair loss most women experience shortly after giving birth. (See **Hair That Isn't There,** above.)

Finally, hair loss in toddlers can also be a telltale sign of various skin diseases, such as bacterial and fungal infections and the dreaded *ringworm* (see **Spotted, Scaly Scalp,** below). These conditions can be highly contagious, and they require treatment with antifungal or antibiotic medications.

SCALP PROBLEMS

MISSING CHUNK OF SCALP SKIN

Q: *My nephew was born with what looks like a small, round, open wound on his scalp. My brother doesn't seem worried, but I am. Could this be a sign of something serious?*

A: It certainly can be disconcerting to see some skin missing from a newborn's head. It may be a sign of *aplasia cutis congenita,* a rare condition in which a baby is born with a piece (or sometimes pieces) of skin missing from the scalp. This is actually a type of *congenital hypotrichosis*. (See **Born Bald,** above.) Although usually found on the back of the head, the raw patch is sometimes seen on the torso, arms, or legs. As scary as it looks and sounds, aplasia cutis congenita is more a cosmetic concern than a medical problem.

It's not known how often aplasia cutis congenita occurs or precisely

---

DANGER SIGN

A ring of long, dark, thick, and rough hair around a cystlike lump can be an early, subtle sign of a *neural tube defect,* a birth defect in which a baby's spinal cord didn't fully develop in the womb. Known as the *hair collar sign,* it's usually seen on the top of the head. It can also be associated with other neurological problems as well as hand deformities.

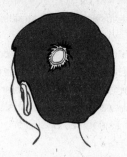

APLASIA CUTIS CONGENITA

what causes it. It's not, however, due to any injury during delivery. In very rare cases children with this condition will have serious medical problems or more obvious physical abnormalities.

Treatment is aimed at preventing bleeding and infections. If small, the wound will probably scab over and new skin will grow in a few weeks. If large, surgery may be needed to close it. Regardless of the size, hair won't grow on the bare spot. But the surrounding head hair can help camouflage it.

SOFT LUMP ON SCALP

Q: *I freaked out when my grandson was born with an ugly lump on his head. What does it mean and will it go away?*

A: It sounds like you're describing what's commonly called a "goose egg." However disconcerting this lump looks, it's probably nothing to worry about. A soft lump on the scalp is usually a harmless *hematoma* (collection of blood), medically known as a *cephalohematoma*. These head bruises occur in approximately 3% of births, and like any bruise, are usually a sign that some small blood vessels leaked under the skin—not inside the skull. They're usually the result of a superficial injury to the baby's head during labor or delivery. It's not surprising, then, that they're often seen on babies delivered by vacuum extraction or forceps. A baby who has a large head or who has a mother with a small pelvis has an increased likelihood of being born with a goose egg.

The goose egg may grow during the baby's first week, but it usually disappears on its own in a few weeks or months. In the past, doctors lanced them, but this treatment often led to infections; so today, they're largely left alone.

If, however, a goose egg or other lump pops up on a baby's head during infancy or toddlerhood, it can be a warning sign of a head injury from an accident, head banging (see Chapter 1), or even abuse. Because any blow to the head can have serious consequences, the baby should be checked out as soon as possible.

WHITE FLAKES ON THE SCALP

Q: *I babysit for a 3-month-old girl whose scalp and hair seem to be sprinkled with flakes. Can it be dandruff?*

A: In a manner of speaking, yes, it can be dandruff. It sounds like you're describing the classic sign of *cradle cap,* medically known as *infantile seborrheic dermatitis* and commonly called "baby dandruff."

Another easily spotted sign of cradle cap is a scalp rash that's yellow or brownish, crusty, greasy, or scaly. Sometimes the crusty patches may also appear on the baby's ears, eyebrows, eyelashes, or face, or even in the armpits and other skin creases.

Cradle cap isn't a sign of poor hygiene. It is usually caused by a combination of oil secretions from *sebaceous glands* (the fat-producing glands) and a yeast or other type of infection.

Luckily, cradle cap is an inconsequential condition. It's most common in the first few months of life and usually clears on its own by the time the baby is 6 to 12 months old. In rare instances, it can linger for longer. You'll be relieved to know that it's not contagious and that it usually doesn't bother the baby (although if it gets really severe, it might itch). It's usually successfully treated with antidandruff shampoos and antifungal lotions and/or ointments.

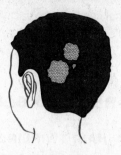

RINGWORM

SPOTTED, SCALY SCALP

Q: Our 15-month-old son's scalp looks like it has little black dots on it. And some of his hair is missing. Could he have picked up a bug at day care?

A: Your baby may be displaying the aptly named *black dot sign,* a hallmark of the common, uncomely condition *ringworm* (aka *tinea capitis*). The black dots are neither bugs nor worms. Rather, they're short stubs of broken hair. These black dots should not be confused with the broken hairs, called *exclamation marks,* which are found at the edges of the bald spots of *alopecia areata* (see **Balding Baby,** above).

Ringworm is a contagious fungal infection that primarily affects the scalp. (It does occur on other parts of the body, but usually in older children and adults.) It weakens the hair structure, which causes the hair to break. The result: The top of the baby's scalp has a "salt-and-pepper" appearance—making the short hairs look like black dots on the skin, which may be difficult to see on children with dark skin.

Other common signs of ringworm are a red, flaky, scaly, or itchy scalp. In severe cases a baby with this condition will develop large, red, spongy, pus-filled swellings on the scalp called *kerions,* which can result in permanent scarring and bald spots.

WARNING SIGN

 Because ringworm is so contagious, siblings and playmates who come in close physical contact with babies with this fungal infection can catch it by sharing toys or personal objects including combs and hairbrushes.

The good news is that ringworm isn't as widespread as it once was. The bad news is that it's highly contagious and, while treatable, can be difficult to get rid of.

HAIR-RELATED BEHAVIOR

HAIR TWIRLING

Q: *Our 1-year-old daughter has been twirling her hair a lot. We've begun to see patches of missing hair on her scalp. Is it just a phase?*

A: While hair twirling may not be as common as thumb sucking, many babies twirl their hair while calmly sucking a bottle or breast-feeding, or while falling asleep. The repetitive motion of hair twirling helps these babies relax. (In fact, even some adults twirl their hair during times of stress.) You may notice that your baby also twists your hair when you hold her. Fortunately, hair twirling is generally a harmless habit, and most children outgrow it.

But hair twirling can lead to a type of hair loss medically known as *trichotillomania,* which involves the pulling or plucking out of hair. It's occasionally mistaken for *alopecia areata* (see **Balding Baby,** above), but the distinguishing sign of trichotillomania is that there are irregular patches of broken hairs, often of differing lengths, rather than a bald patch. These patches are often found on one side of the head—the one closest to the baby's dominant hand—and only in areas within the baby's reach. Some children will pull hairs from the crown of the head, which leads to the distinctive and descriptive *Friar Tuck sign.* Children have been known to pull out not only their scalp hair but also their eyebrows and eyelashes. Trichotillomania is much more common in girls than boys and can run in families.

Although trichotillomania can sometimes cause Mom and Dad to pull out their own hair, it doesn't cause damage to the hair follicles or permanent loss of hair. But there's some debate about whether trichotillomania that starts in infancy is a habit or an early sign of *obsessive-compulsive disorder* (*OCD*) or another underlying behavioral problem, such as anxiety.

A small number of children who pull out their hair will also eat it, a be-

WARNING SIGN

Pulling out and eating dolls' hair can be an early sign of trichotillomania and trichophagia.

havioral disorder known as *trichophagia*. This is a form of *pica,* a condition in which a person habitually eats nonfood items, such as clay and paint chips. (They may even eat their mothers' hair.) In rare cases, these children can actually develop hairballs—a condition called *Rapunzel syndrome*. The hairballs usually need to be removed surgically.

SIGNING OFF

During a newborn's physical examination, the baby's head and body will be checked for any unusual color or patches of hair. Because many hair signs of medical problems don't become apparent until later—when most babies grow hair—parents are often the first to notice them.

NOTIFY YOUR CHILD'S HEALTHCARE PROVIDER IF:
- Your baby's hair is very hard to comb or breaks or falls out when you comb it.
- A change in your baby's hair is accompanied by a skin change—one that looks like an inflammation or infection, or skin that bleeds, oozes, scabs over, or itches.
- There is any change in the amount, color, or texture of your baby's hair.

While a pediatrician can often diagnose and treat the underlying cause of many hair-related illnesses, a specialist may sometimes be needed. Dermatologists and endocrinologists are often called in to evaluate and manage some cases.

CHAPTER 3

YOUR BABY'S EYES

Here are my eyes,
One and two.
I give a wink.
So can you.
When they are open,
I see the light.
When they are closed
It's dark like night.
—Traditional nursery rhyme

PROBABLY ONE OF THE MOST unforgettable and rewarding moments new parents experience is when their baby first glances into their eyes. Many newborns open their eyes a few minutes after birth and look around, checking out the outside world and, more important, their parents. Although it may take a while before they're able to focus well enough to look directly into their parents' eyes, by the 3rd month most babies can zero in on any object.

For parents, babies' eyes are the windows to their emotions, if not their very souls. And a glance into a baby's eyes can give both parents and physicians key information about the baby's health. Indeed, eyes are the

SIGNIFICANT FACT

⚠ Vision is the last sense to develop both inside and outside the womb.

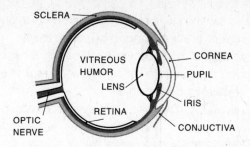

SCLERA

VITREOUS
HUMOR

LENS

RETINA

OPTIC
NERVE

CORNEA

PUPIL

IRIS

CONJUCTIVA

EYE ANATOMY

focal point of many body signs found in infants and adults alike. These signs may be read in a baby's eye color, pupils, movement, and even tears.

EYE COLOR SIGNS

Like the color of our hair, the color of our eyes is determined by our genes. Most babies are born with blue or gray eyes, which slowly darken over the next 3 to 6 months, some ultimately turning brown.

DIFFERENT-COLORED EYES

Q: Our adopted baby has one brown and one blue eye. Is this something he inherited, and could there be something wrong with him?

A: Having different-colored eyes—medically known as *heterochromia*—is a rare condition in which a person has two different-colored irises. (There is another, less common form of this condition in which one iris can be two different colors, creating a piebald or mottled effect.)

Heterochromia is usually a benign, inherited trait. It can be present at birth (congenital) or be acquired at any age as a result of a serious eye infection or physical injury to the eye.

However, if a baby has different-colored eyes as well as a streak of white hair or a white forelock, it can signal *Waardenburg syndrome* (see Chapter 2), a rare, potentially serious, genetic condition. Children with this disorder often suffer from vision problems and deafness. Although there's no cure, vision and hearing problems can usually be treated, allowing the children to lead normal lives.

Heterochromia can be a sign of several other congenital, but not inherited, conditions, including *Duane syndrome,* an eye-movement disorder that sometimes also affects a child's vision (See **An Up-Cast Eye,** below) and congenital *Horner's syndrome,* a nerve disorder. Other common signs of Horner's include two different-sized pupils and a droopy eyelid. (See **Mismatched Pupils** and **Droopy Eyes,** below.) Facial sweating on the affected side is sometimes absent.

> ## SIGN OF THE TIMES
>
> The ancient Greeks feared people with blue eyes, believing they could cast the evil eye upon enemies. To ward off this threat, they carried around blue charms that looked like blue eyes. Today, many Greeks—as well as other southern Europeans and Middle Easterners—still carry these blue amulets.

> ## SIGN OF THE TIMES
>
> Aristotle, Alexander the Great, and Louis Pasteur were reported to have two different-colored eyes. Some modern-day celebrities—including Kate Bosworth, Jane Seymour, Kiefer Sutherland, and Christopher Walken—do as well.

PALE OR PINK EYES

Q: *My 2-month-old niece, who has very pale blue eyes, was diagnosed with albinism. Don't albinos have pink eyes? If she is an albino, will her vision be affected?*

A: While most people with albinism do have pink eyes, some have very light blue or gray eyes. Albinism is a rare genetic disorder in which the body doesn't produce an adequate amount of melanin, the substance responsible for eye, skin, and hair color. In addition to pink or pale eyes, babies and children with this condition often have very fair skin and white or yellowish hair (see Chapter 2).

STOP SIGN

(STOP) Babies' eyes—especially light-colored eyes—are very sun-sensitive. So make sure that your baby wears a hat or sunglasses whenever he or she is out in the sun.

Most children with albinism do suffer from eye problems such as poor vision, light sensitivity, crossed eyes, and *nystagmus,* which is rapid, uncontrollable back-and-forth or up-and-down eye movements (see **Unusual Eye Movements and Positions,** below). In some cases, albinism is also associated with deafness.

With the exception of these eye problems, most albinos are healthy. They do, however, have to be very careful in the sun because they're at increased risk for serious sunburn and, as a result, skin cancer. There is no cure for albinism; treatment focuses on correcting a child's vision and other eye problems.

SIGN OF THE TIMES

Charles Darwin was one of the first scientists to note the connection between albinism and deafness . . . at least in cats. More recently, scientists have found that in certain ethnic groups, most notably the Hopi Indians in the United States, the incidence of albinism and deafness is exceedingly high, affecting 1 in 200 people.

RED EYES

Q: *The whites of our newborn's eyes are bright red. Could he have an eye infection?*

A: Your baby may have a condition commonly seen in newborns called *subconjunctival hemorrhage.* It's usually the result of a mild trauma to the baby's eye or eyes during birth. The hemorrhage is like a red black-and-blue mark and is caused by blood leaking under the thin membrane covering the eyeball. Like other bruises, it will usually fade in a few days.

However, if the whites of a baby's eyes remain red or look irritated, it can be a sign of an allergy, or *pinkeye,* a highly contagious eye infection medically known as *conjunctivitis.* The affected eye or eyes of a child with pinkeye may be crusty and stuck shut in the morning. Even if only one eye is infected, it's likely to spread to the other eye (and to other people) unless immediately treated.

YELLOW EYES

Q: The whites of our newborn's eyes have recently turned yellow. Could he have jaundice? And isn't jaundice a sign of liver disease?

A: Indeed, yellow eyes can be a telltale sign of jaundice, which is very common in infants. In fact, more than half of all newborns have what's called *physiologic jaundice,* which can also turn their skin yellow. This is usually a temporary, benign condition unrelated to liver or other diseases.

Jaundice is the result of a buildup of *bilirubin,* a yellow-orange substance produced by the breakdown of red blood cells. Because their immature livers can't process the bilirubin fast enough, many newborns wind up with yellow eyes and/or skin. The good news is that in most cases the jaundice usually disappears in about a week.

WARNING SIGN

Jaundiced eyes in babies of African descent can be an important warning sign of *sickle-cell anemia*. Jaundiced skin may be more difficult to detect in some children with dark skin.

But yellow eyes (and skin) that persist past the first week of life can be signs of *breast milk jaundice*, a usually harmless condition in which certain substances in breast milk interfere with the breakdown of bilirubin. This type of jaundice, which may last 6 weeks or longer, tends to run in families. Although usually nothing to worry about, babies with breast milk jaundice need to be carefully evaluated and their bilirubin levels measured.

Jaundice in an infant can also be a warning sign that the baby is not getting enough breast milk—medically known as *breast-feeding jaundice.* (This should not be confused with *breast milk jaundice,* which is usually benign.) In breast-feeding jaundice, the baby's bilirubin level may become too high, which can cause liver damage and other serious problems. Treatment usually involves phototherapy (light therapy) and more frequent nursing. In very severe cases of breast-feeding jaundice, supplemental feeding with formula may be required.

In some babies, jaundice may be a warning sign of an infection or thyroid problem, both of which require treatment. It can also signal *Rh disease,* a blood-type incompatibility, which is

> ### SIGNIFICANT FACT
>
> Because bilirubin is excreted in bowel movements, babies with jaundice have pale poop. So the more these babies poop, the faster their skin and their poop will regain normal color.

potentially life threatening to both the mother and infant. In most cases, Rh incompatibility is preventable with prenatal and postnatal treatment of the mother. Without treatment, babies born with Rh disease (aka *hemolytic disease of the newborn*) may suffer from a variety of complications that can range in severity from mild anemia and jaundice to severe anemia, brain damage, and even heart failure.

Regardless of the cause of jaundice, when a baby's eyes or skin remain yellow for more than a few weeks, bilirubin levels need to be measured. If they are high, prompt treatment is necessary to prevent such serious disorders as liver disease, deafness, cerebral palsy, and even brain damage. Treatment usually involves phototherapy, but in very rare cases an exchange blood transfusion may be necessary.

"WHITE EYE" IN PHOTOS

Q: I heard that red-eye in a photograph is a good sign, but if a baby's eyes have a white dot in photos, it's considered a bad sign. Is this true?

A: Red-eye in a photograph is, indeed, regarded as a healthy sign. Known as the *red reflex,* it's caused by the camera's flash lighting up the blood-rich retina at the back of the eyes. However, when an eye looks white instead of red in a photo, it's an important warning sign that something is blocking the retina. Medically known as *leukocoria,* which literally means "white pupil," it usually affects only one eye and covers most, if not all, of the pupil. Besides being visible in photographs, the *white reflex,* as it's also called, can sometimes be spotted in dim light. It can make a child's eye shine like a cat's eye at night. In fact, this reaction is aptly named the *cat's eye reflex.*

The single white spot of leukocoria should *not* be confused with the smaller white dots that appear in *both* eyes in photographs. Like red-eye, these dots are seen in the same position in each eye and are a normal photographic phenomenon of light bouncing off the cornea, which is in the front of the eye.

WARNING SIGN

While having the white-eye reflex is usually proof positive of a serious eye problem, having red-eye in a photograph doesn't necessarily rule out serious eye disease.

Leukocoria is a red flag for several serious eye disorders including cataracts, retinal detachments, and infections inside the eye. It's also the most common warning sign of *retinoblastoma,* a very rare and serious childhood cancer. Genetic but not always inherited, this cancer primarily affects babies between infancy and 2 years of age. Other common signs of retinoblastoma are crossed or misaligned eyes (see **Crossed Eyes,** below); a red, swollen eye; and what some parents describe as "a white, shiny, Jell-O-like eye." In most cases, it occurs in only one eye. When it affects both eyes, it's virtually always inherited.

STOP SIGN

 It's very important to occasionally have your baby's photo taken *without* the "red-eye reduction" camera feature. This can help rule out retinal disease.

The average baby with retinoblastoma is diagnosed at 18 months, and most cases are first recognized by parents rather than doctors. Unfortunately, even when parents notice the telltale warning signs, they may not mention it to their baby's doctor, which can result in delayed diagnosis and treatment. Without prompt medical intervention, this cancer is life threatening. Although treatment may occasionally involve the loss of an eye, most children have 20/20 vision in the remaining eye. And the cancer is totally curable in 95% of cases when caught and treated early.

"YELLOW-EYE" IN PHOTOS

Q: *I've noticed that one of my son's eyes usually looks yellow in photographs. Can there be something seriously wrong with his eye?*

A: When an eye looks yellow in a photograph, which is referred to as *yellow-eye reflex,* it may be a telltale sign of *Coats' disease,* a very serious, rare genetic eye disorder. Coats' disease affects the retina and is often mistaken for retinoblastoma, an eye cancer found in children (see **"White Eye" in Photos,** above). Although Coats' is not a cancer, it's a progressive disease that can cause partial or even complete blindness. It occurs mostly in young boys under age 10, and usually affects only one eye. If they're old enough to express themselves, children with Coats' disease may complain of vision problems.

Treatment may involve laser surgery or cryotherapy (freezing). In severe cases, surgical removal of the eye may be necessary. In some cases, however, Coats' stops progressing on its own, and there have even been documented cases of spontaneous cures.

MISMATCHED PUPILS

Q: *One of my daughter's pupils is bigger than the other. Why is that and should I be concerned?*

A: Having different-sized pupils, medically known as *anisocoria,* is an often benign, surprisingly common inherited trait. In fact, 1 in 5 people have one pupil that's smaller than the other, and most are born that way. When mismatched pupils are present at birth, they are usually nothing to worry about, especially if there are no other unusual signs. Anisocoria can also occur anytime after birth, usually as the result of an eye infection or injury. In these cases, the child should be carefully evaluated for other problems.

SIGNIFICANT FACT

People with blue eyes tend to have larger pupils than those with brown eyes.

Different-sized pupils along with two different-colored eyes and/or a droopy eyelid may be a sign of *congenital Horner's syndrome* (see **Different-Colored Eyes,** above, and **Droopy Eyes,** below), which is usually a benign condition. But Horner's can also develop at any age, usually as a result of an injury to the neck, eye, facial nerves, spinal cord, or brain.

WARNING SIGN

Acquired Horner's can be the earliest warning sign of *neuroblastoma,* a rare, fast-growing, malignant tumor, which occurs most often in the abdomen. Neuroblastoma is by far the most common cancer in infants. In most cases, unfortunately, the cancer is not diagnosed until it has metastasized (spread). The good news is that when caught early, it's usually successfully treated with surgery and/or chemotherapy. The even better news is that in about 1 in 3 cases of neuroblastoma, the cancer will disappear spontaneously if the tumor hasn't already spread.

When anisocoria occurs very suddenly, it can be a danger sign of a life-threatening condition such as a cerebral hemorrhage, an aneurysm, a brain tumor, meningitis, or encephalitis.

MISSHAPEN PUPIL

Q: The pupil of one of our son's eyes is oval rather than round. Can this affect his vision?

DANGER SIGNS

Seek immediate medical attention if you notice that your baby has suddenly acquired mismatched pupils and:

- It follows an eye or head injury.
- It's accompanied by vomiting or a fever.
- Your baby becomes light-sensitive or seems like he or she is having trouble seeing.
- Your baby appears to have head, eye, or neck pain.

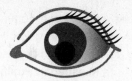

IRIS COLOBOMA

A: It sounds like your son might have a relatively rare eye abnormality known as *iris coloboma,* which can occur in one or both eyes. Although the defect is in the iris and not the pupil, the pupil often looks like an old-fashioned keyhole or has some other unusual shape. Sometimes the flaw in the iris is so close to the pupil that the pupil itself looks like it's split. It can also look like there's a hole in the iris.

Most colobomas are congenital and are noticed at or shortly after birth. They're usually the result of incomplete eye development during early pregnancy. In fact, *coloboma* comes from the Greek word for "unfinished."

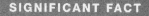
SIGNIFICANT FACT

 The word *iris* comes from the Latin word for "rainbow."

If a child is born with iris coloboma, it's most likely a benign, cosmetic condition. But a coloboma can sometimes cause blurred vision and light sensitivity, particularly if it extends into the eye itself.

In very rare cases, a child with a coloboma may have a genetic condition such as *cat eye syndrome,* which is associated with other more obvious facial deformities and serious intestinal, kidney, and heart problems.

SIGNIFICANT FACT

Some older children and adults who have colobomas choose to wear colored contact lenses to mask their unusual eyes.

DOUBLE PUPIL

Q: My granddaughter looks like she has two pupils in one eye. Can she see normally through that eye?

A: Two pupils in one eye is medically known as *polycoria* (aka *dicoria* or *diplocoria*), a rare congenital condition that is actually a type of coloboma (see **Misshapen Pupil,** above). While the extra pupil usually doesn't function, there have been a few reported cases in which the second pupil contracts like a normal one. Fortunately, the double pupils themselves don't usually interfere with vision. However, as with other forms of colobomas, multiple pupils can be associated with vision and other medical problems (see **Misshapen Pupil,** above).

EYELID PROBLEMS

RED EYELIDS

Q: Our 1-year-old daughter has one red, swollen eyelid. What can cause this?

A: Your daughter may have gotten an insect bite or suffered an injury to that eye. However, there's a chance that she may have a bacterial eye infection called *preseptal cellulitis,* a condition that can be caused by an insect bite. It usually affects only one eye. Other signs may include a runny nose, a fever, or conjunctivitis (see **Red Eyes,** above). If your daughter's eyeball is also swollen, it can signal a more severe infection called *orbital cellulitis*. Both of these infections can usually be treated easily with antibiotics when caught early. Without treatment, however, they can cause serious eye problems including blindness, and may also lead to meningitis or other life-threatening disorders.

CRUSTY EYELIDS

Q: My 6-month-old son's eyelids are crusty and look irritated. What could it be?

A: Crusty eyelids are the hallmark of a fairly common condition called *blepharitis* (aka *granulated eyelids*), an inflammation at the base of the eyelashes that often affects both eyes. Other signs may include teary, itchy eyes, red-rimmed eyelids, and matted eyelashes. In some cases, the eyelashes may even temporarily fall out.

Most cases of blepharitis are caused by either the *staphylococcus* bacteria or by *seborrheic dermatitis,* which also causes dandruff and cradle cap (see Chapter 2). But in rare cases, it may be a warning sign of lice on the eyelid.

While blepharitis doesn't usually affect vision, it can lead to conjunctivitis (see **Red Eyes,** above) or other serious eye infections if left untreated. Treatment typically involves antibiotic ointments or drops, warm compresses, and gentle washing of eyelids. But even when it's treated successfully, blepharitis often recurs throughout childhood and even into adulthood.

EYELID LUMP OR BUMP

Q: Our infant daughter has a tiny lump on her eyelid that looks like a sty. Can it be?

A: If the bump is near the eyelashes, it could be a *sty* (also spelled *stye*). Medically known as a *hordeolum,* a sty is actually a tiny pimple. It's caused by an infection in a *sebaceous* (oil) gland, which sits at the base of the eyelashes. Like larger pimples, sties are usually red, inflamed, and may be filled with pus. They'll often rupture in 2 to 4 days, causing your baby's eyelid to look crusty. But if the lump grows, your daughter may have a *chalazion*—a blocked oil gland. Several of them may pop up on the same eyelid.

Although the terms *sty* and *chalazion* are sometimes used interchangeably, they are, in fact, different conditions. While sties are due to an acute infection, chalazions are caused by the blockage of a sweat gland in the eyelid, which can become infected if left untreated. Chalazions also tend to last longer than sties, usually 1 to 3 months. And they're usually larger, growing to the size of a pea or even a marble. Some grow so large that they press on a child's eyeball, distorting vision.

Although both sties and chalazions are typically benign, they should be treated in order to prevent a more serious infection. Simple mea-

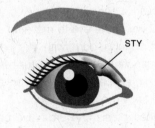
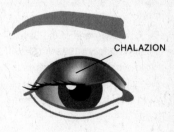

STY **CHALAZION**

sures such as warm compresses are usually recommended, but in some cases antibiotic drops or ointments are needed. Although the lumps may disappear with treatment, they can recur.

DROOPY EYES

Q: My baby girl has droopy eyelids. No one else in the family does. What could have caused this?

A: Eyelid droop is medically known as *ptosis*. It may affect one or both eyes and it can either be present at birth or show up later in life. In a newborn, droopy eyes may be a perfectly normal facial feature. But ptosis, especially in one eye, can be a telltale sign of the nerve disorder *Horner's syndrome* (see **Different-Colored Eyes** and **Mismatched Pupils,** above).

Droopy eyes can also signal *congenital myasthenia gravis* (*MG*), an inherited disorder. (This is different from the MG seen in adulthood, which is an autoimmune disease.) It causes muscle weakness in various parts of the body, especially the arms and legs, which can result in delayed motor skills. Babies with congenital MG often have poor head control and difficulty feeding. Although it's a chronic condition, treatment with medication often helps.

Ptosis in a newborn can also signal *3rd-nerve palsy,* a weakness of the 3rd cranial nerve that interferes with the ability of the eye to move up and down. Babies born with this nerve disorder often have had difficult births. Over time, the nerve condition and the droopy eye may clear up.

When ptosis and 3rd-nerve palsy occur after birth, they may be due to

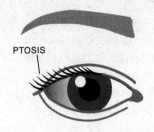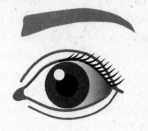

PTOSIS

PTOSIS (DROOPY EYELID)

physical trauma to the head. In rare cases, the ptosis and palsy may be due to a serious infection such as meningitis, or, very rarely, a brain tumor. In these instances, however, the child would have more severe and obvious signs than a droopy eye.

Regardless of the cause, babies with ptosis are at increased risk of developing *amblyopia,* a condition in which a normal (healthy) eye loses vision, and *astigmatism,* an eye defect that causes images to look distorted or blurred. Depending on how much the droopy eyelid affects a child's vision and/or physical appearance, surgery may be needed. Because ptosis is often permanent, it's important to treat not only the underlying cause but the physical and social consequences as well.

WARNING SIGN

 One eyelid that suddenly droops may be a warning sign that your baby has a serious infection or tumor. In some cases, it can also signal a stroke.

DOUBLE EYELASHES

Q: Our daughter has 2 rows of eyelashes. They make her eyes look beautiful, but are they normal?

A: It sounds like your daughter has what's medically known as *distichiasis.* In this rare, usually inherited condition, 2 hairs grow out of a single

SPEAKING OF SIGNS

The slime of snails, applied of the eyes of children, straightens the eyelashes, and makes them grow.
—Pliny the Elder (A.D. 23–79), Roman historian, *Natural History Book*

follicle. There may be a whole row of double lashes or just a few. While these double lashes make the eyes look exotic, they can be problematic. The extra lashes can grow toward the cornea, scratching and irritating it. This may result in chronic abrasions or eye ulcers.

Double eyelashes can also be a very early warning sign of the genetic condition *lymphedema-distichiasis syndrome,* which causes tissue swelling (*edema*) primarily in the legs and feet. The swelling, which doesn't usually occur until late childhood or puberty, tends to affect boys sooner than girls. Other eye problems seen in children with this chronic condition include ptosis (see **Droopy Eyes,** above), light sensitivity, and repeated bouts of conjunctivitis and sties (see **Red Eyes** and **Eyelid Lump or Bump,** above). Some children with lymphedema-distichiasis syndrome may also have a congenital heart defect or other anatomic abnormalities and may be at increased risk for early-onset varicose veins. Although lymphedema-distichiasis is a chronic condition, there are effective treatments for the edema and/or eye problems.

Whether the distichiasis is related to lymphedema or not, babies with double eyelashes must have their eyes monitored for eye abrasions. In some cases, extra lashes may need to be removed to reduce the risk of eye irritations, infections, and other complications.

WARNING SIGN

Because the swelling of lymphedema usually doesn't show up until late childhood or puberty, all children with double eyelashes should undergo genetic testing. If they have the gene marker for lymphedema, further medical evaluation is needed to rule out cardiac or other serious problems. Family members should consider genetic testing as well.

CIRCLES, BAGS, AND BULGES

BABY SHINERS

Q: I heard that dark circles around a baby's eyes may signal allergies rather than a lack of sleep. Is that true?

A: It's true: Lack of sleep isn't a major cause of eye circles or bags in babies, but allergies are. In fact, they're commonly referred to as "allergic shiners" and are especially common in *atopic* children—that is, children who have an inherited tendency to develop allergies.

Dark circles can also signal sinus infections and other nasal problems that cause congestion. In these conditions, the veins around the eyes become blocked and engorged, resulting in the dark circles and sometimes bags. When the allergy or nasal problem is treated successfully, the circles often fade.

Dark circles can also be an inherited trait unrelated to allergies or other problems, and are especially noticeable in children who have fair complexions. In these cases, they're unlikely to fade.

BABY BAGS

Q: *What does it mean when a baby is born with bags or skin folds under the eyes?*

A: Bags or skin folds under a newborn's eyes may be an inherited trait called *Dennie-Morgan lines*. Also called Denni-Morgan or Denny-Morgan skin folds, they're similar to allergic shiners (see **Baby Shiners,** above), but they're permanent. Indeed, fully 60% to 80% of atopic children (see **Baby Shiners,** above) have these lines. Children with Dennie-Morgan skin folds are at increased risk not only for serious allergies but for asthma as well.

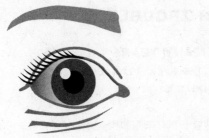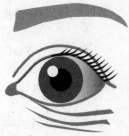

DENNIE-MORGAN SKIN FOLDS

PROTRUDING EYES

Q: *My toddler son's eyes are so large that they seem to bulge out of his head. Besides not liking the way it looks, I'm worried that something is wrong. Should I be?*

A: Bulging eyes, medically known as *proptosis* or *exophthalmos,* can be a normal, inherited trait or a sign of several medical conditions. If both of your son's eyes protrude, he may have *Graves' disease,* the most common form of *hyperthyroidism,* an overactive thyroid gland. Other signs include excessive hunger, weight loss, fast pulse, nervousness, and irritability. Graves' disease is usually treated with medicine and in very rare cases surgery.

Bulging or very large eyes can also signal a rare, potentially serious condition, *infantile glaucoma* (aka *primary congenital glaucoma*). Although babies with this disorder are born with it, it may go unnoticed for several months. This form of glaucoma occurs more often in boys than girls, and usually affects both eyes. Other common signs include light sensitivity, eyelid spasms, and excessive tearing. The child's eyes may also look cloudy or hazy. If untreated, congenital glaucoma can damage the optic nerve, leading to blindness. Surgery is usually needed to correct this condition.

STOP SIGN

(STOP) Anyone who's had congenital glaucoma—even after treatment—should have their eyes carefully checked throughout their lives. Glaucoma can recur at any age, threatening vision.

TEAR TROUBLE

TOO MANY TEARS

Q: My baby boy's eyes are often teary. And when he cries, rivers of tears stream out. What could be causing this?

A: Your son's excessive tearing—medically known as *epiphora*—may be the result of an allergy or eye irritation. Or it may be a warning sign of congenital glaucoma (see **Protruding Eyes,** above).

Overflowing tears are also a classic sign of a blocked tear duct (aka *dacryostenosis*), a very common condition in infants. Tears are produced in the *lacrimal gland,* above the outer eyelashes and below the eyebrow. They then flow over the eyeball and enter the *puncta* (a tiny opening in the corner of the eye), the *lacrimal sac,* and finally the tear

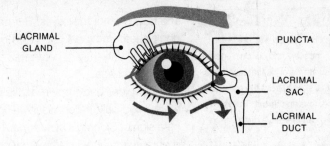

LACRIMAL (TEAR) SYSTEM

duct (aka *nasolacrimal duct*). If the duct is blocked, the tears back up, overflow, and stream down the face (much the way a clogged sink overflows). This can happen in one or both eyes. Yellow mucus can also build up in the corner of the eye, causing the eye to become crusty and irritated.

A blocked tear duct may result from a structural problem or an infection. A blockage can also cause a serious infection in the tear duct system. Fortunately, about 9 in 10 cases of blocked tear ducts clear up on their own by the time a baby is a year old. Simple measures, such as massage or warm compresses, tend to work. Sometimes a minor surgical procedure is needed to open a blocked duct.

SIGNIFICANT FACT

There are two kinds of tears—those that lubricate the eye, and those that are a reaction to pain or emotion. And scientists have recently discovered that the two kinds have different chemical compositions. Emotional tears contain more protein and stress-related hormones than the tears that bathe the eyes.

NO TEARS

Q: Our 2-month-old daughter cries a lot but she doesn't have any tears. Could she possibly have a blocked tear duct?

A: It's unlikely that your daughter has a blocked tear duct because babies with this condition actually do produce tears. (See **Too Many Tears,** above.) Your daughter, like most newborns, is probably tearless because her tear system has not yet fully developed. By the end of the first month, most babies produce *basal tears,* which lubricate, cleanse,

The reason why our babies' noses—and our own—tend to run when we cry is that tear ducts carry tears away from the eyes and into the nose and throat. This is also why we can taste eye drops.

and help protect their eyes. But most don't shed emotional tears (aka *psychic tears*) until they're between 2 and 4 months of age.

In an older baby, however, lack of tears, medically called *alacrima,* can be a sign of *Sjögren's syndrome*. This is an autoimmune, inflammatory condition that damages the moisture-producing glands, causing dryness of the eyes, nose, and skin. Other parts of the body, including the internal organs, can be affected as well. While fairly common in adults, Sjögren's is quite rare in children. Whether in children or adults, it's primarily seen in females. Although there's no cure for Sjögren's, medicines can treat the dryness and other problems it causes, and help prevent further complications.

DANGER SIGN

If your baby suddenly stops producing tears and has scanty or dark urine, and possibly sunken eyes, he or she may be dangerously dehydrated. Take your baby to the emergency room immediately.

Lack of tears is also the hallmark of *familial dysautonomia* (*FD*), a rare genetic condition that primarily affects Jews of Eastern European (Ashkenazi) descent.

In this inherited condition, the autonomic and sensory nervous systems—the ones that control such vital functions as heart rate, blood pressure, breathing, and body temperature—don't function properly. In addition to a lack of tears, other signs of FD may include a weak sucking reflex, blotchy skin, difficulty maintaining normal body temperature, and poor muscle tone. As children with this condition grow older, they may experience a whole range of sensory and other medical problems.

For unknown reasons, many children with familial dysautonomia were breech births.

Although they usually have normal intelligence, they may be at increased risk for learning disabilities. While familial dysautonomia is not curable, most problems caused by this disorder can be treated medically.

HAPPY TEARS

Q: *When my baby nurses, his tears flow, even though he seems very happy. Are these tears of joy or tears of pain?*

A: Your son may be displaying the signs of a very rare phenomenon aptly called *crocodile tear(s) syndrome* (aka *gustatory hyperlacrimation*). Babies with this syndrome start crying as soon as they begin to nurse or drink from a bottle. While usually benign, this condition can be associated with *Duane syndrome,* an eye movement disorder (see **An Up-Cast Eye,** below).

Most children with crocodile tear syndrome are born with it. But some develop it after an eye infection, physical trauma, or *Bell's palsy,* a usually benign nerve disorder that causes temporary facial weakness or paralysis.

For the most part, crocodile tear syndrome doesn't need treatment. But in severe cases, medicine or surgery may be recommended.

> ### SIGN OF THE TIMES
>
> The term *crying crocodile tears* refers to insincere or false tears and dates back at least to the 13th century. It was a French myth that crocodiles shed tears while eating their human victims in a show of fake remorse. These cold-blooded creatures actually do produce and shed tears, but they're for lubrication, not fabrication.

UNUSUAL EYE MOVEMENTS AND POSITIONS

DARTING EYES

Q: *Our son's eyes sometimes move quickly from side to side. Is this something to worry about?*

A: It sounds as if your son has the classic sign of *nystagmus,* an eye disorder involving jerky, involuntary eye movements. One or both eyes may move rapidly back and forth, up and down, or around in circles. These eye movements may be constant or sporadic, lasting anywhere from a few minutes to several hours.

If your son was born with this condition, or developed it within the first few months of life, he most likely has what's referred to as *congen-*

SIGNIFICANT FACTS

Most children with albinism have nystagmus. But it's usually not noticed until a child is 2 months old. In fact, nystagmus can signal *ocular albinism,* a rare form of albinism in which the child (or adult) does not have the typical pale eyes and skin.

SIGN OF THE TIMES

Achromatopsia was a little-known eye disorder until 1966, the year the noted neurologist and author Dr. Oliver Sacks published a book about it called *The Island of the Colorblind.* This bestseller was about a small Micronesian island in which a large percentage of the inhabitants suffer from this very rare, serious eye disease.

ital or *infantile nystagmus.* This sometimes runs in families. Although it often improves by age 5 or 6, congenital or infantile nystagmus is usually a permanent condition. While most cases are benign, some affected babies have or will develop other vision problems or medical conditions.

It can, for example, be the first warning sign of a very rare genetic condition, *achromatopsia,* which is a serious form of color blindness. Most children with this disorder see very little, if any, color; are extremely sensitive to light; and have poor vision.

Nystagmus can be an early sign of *Leber's congenital amaurosis (LCA),* another extremely rare genetic disorder that causes poor vision and severe light sensitivity. Children with LCA sometimes have ear, heart, kidney, neurological, and musculoskeletal abnormalities as well.

If your son developed this eye movement problem *after* infancy (called *acquired nystagmus*), it may signal other eye disorders, including cataracts, glaucoma, and retinal problems. Acquired nystagmus can also occur with *Graves' disease*, an overactive thyroid (see **Protruding Eyes,** above), as well as several

STOP SIGN

Children should be tested for color blindness as early as possible. Since many toys and preschool activities are color dependent, teachers should be alerted if a child is color-blind. Otherwise they may mistakenly think that the child has a language or other problem.

Early detection is also important for safety. A child who is color-blind may not be able to tell the difference between red and green traffic lights.

inner ear disorders. And it can be a very early warning sign of a number of neurological conditions including multiple sclerosis, a brain tumor, or even a stroke. A blow to the head can sometimes cause nystagmus, in which case it may be a warning sign of a brain injury.

CROSSED EYES

Q: *I've heard that babies with crossed eyes often grow out of it. Is that true?*

A: That may be true depending on how young—or old—a baby is when the crossed eyes are first sighted. Eye movement disorders, medically referred to as *strabismus,* are very common in newborns. The majority of these babies have crossed eyes— that is, one eye that turns slightly inward. This condition is medically known as *esotropia.* When it occurs in infancy, babies usually outgrow it by 3 months.

Much rarer, and more serious, is when crossed eyes show up in older babies. When an older baby develops crossed eyes, usually between 2 and 4 months of age, it's referred to as *infantile* or *congenital esotropia.* Babies do *not* outgrow this form of esotropia, which may be inherited. Eye-muscle

> **SIGNIFICANT FACT**
>
> There's a condition called *pseudostrabismus,* in which a baby's eyes look crossed but aren't. It's actually an optical illusion, which can occur when a baby has closely set eyes, a flat nasal bridge, asymmetrical eyelids, or a prominent *epicanthal fold* (the skin fold of the upper eyelid). Although any baby can have a prominent epicanthal fold, they are most commonly seen in Asian babies.

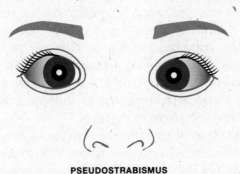

PSEUDOSTRABISMUS

surgery is often recommended, but even then, the condition may recur later in childhood or adulthood, requiring further surgery.

When older babies or toddlers become cross-eyed, it's referred to as *accommodative (refractive) esotropia*. Children with this condition usually have farsighted eyes (*hyperopia*). This type of esotropia tends to affect children between 2 and 3 years old. At first the crossed eyes may be seen only intermittently, but within a few weeks they will constantly turn inward. While children may outgrow accommodative esotropia, prescription eyeglasses can usually correct the problem, prevent vision loss, and decrease the likelihood that surgery is needed. Vision therapy is also sometimes recommended.

STOP SIGN

STOP It's essential that any babies beyond infancy who have strabismus receive early treatment. Without it, they can develop serious vision problems, including vision loss.

AN OUTWARD-DRIFTING EYE

Q: *When she looks straight ahead, my daughter's right eye sometimes turns outward. Will this affect her vision and can it be corrected?*

A: When one eye turns outward, it's medically known as *exotropia* and commonly referred to as a "walleye." This type of strabismus often runs in families and is thought to be caused by eye-muscle weakness. Rarely seen in newborns, it usually first appears in children between 1 and 4 years of age. In most of these children, the eye only occasionally turns out (*intermittent exotropia*), usually when the child is daydreaming, looking at distant objects, or overly tired. The child may also close the weaker eye when under bright lights or out in the sun.

In rare cases, a child's eye will continuously turn out, a condition aptly called *constant exotropia*. Children with constant exotropia sometimes also have medical problems such as neurological disorders, developmental delays, and facial abnormalities.

Without early treatment, children with both types of exotropia can develop serious vision problems, such as loss of depth perception and *amblyopia* (aka "lazy eye"), which is a loss of vision in a healthy eye (see

Droopy Eyes, above). Treatments include eye patches, prescription glasses, and vision therapy. Surgery may be recommended, especially for constant exotropia.

AN UP-CAST EYE

Q: *My newborn niece's right eye sometimes drifts upward, while the left eye looks straight ahead. My sister says it's normal. Is it?*

A: An eye that occasionally turns upward can be a sign of a benign type of *strabismus* (eye misalignment) called *hypertropia*. But it sometimes signals a congenital condition such as *4th-nerve palsy* (aka *superior oblique palsy*). Children with this type of palsy may experience double vision (*diplopia*) and tilt their heads to help them see better.

Although it's not usually associated with other medical problems, hypertropia is a permanent condition. Treatments such as special glasses, vision therapy, and sometimes surgery can help straighten out the eyes.

An up-cast eye can also be a sign of *Duane syndrome* (*DS*), a rare congenital disorder in which one eye has limited ability to move right or left. Instead, the eye tends to move upward, or in some cases, downward. The affected eye may also look smaller than the normal one. As with 4th-nerve palsy, some children tilt their heads to help align their eyes. This eye-muscle disorder is thought to occur during the 6th week of pregnancy as a result of both genetic and environmental factors in the womb.

Duane syndrome is more common in girls than in boys. It tends to affect the left eye, but sometimes it occurs in both eyes. It's not usually associated with any serious medical disorders, but some children with DS may have cataracts, reduced vision in the affected eye, nystagmus (see **Darting Eyes,** above), crocodile tear syndrome (see **Happy**

Tears, above), and other eye problems. And in rare cases children with DS may have ear, kidney, nervous system, or skeletal abnormalities. While any serious underlying condition must be treated, DS is primarily a cosmetic problem that doesn't require treatment. However, in severe cases, surgery may be recommended.

ANGELIC EYES

Q: Our newly adopted son's eyes sometimes gaze upward for several hours at a time. While this makes him look angelic, should we be concerned?

A: Upward-gazing eyes can be a sign of a rare condition called *benign paroxysmal tonic upgaze* (*PTU*). It's usually first noticed when a child is under a year old, and it sometimes runs in families.

Although it's often preceded by a fever or infection, PTU is usually a benign condition, as the name implies. However, some children with PTU have mild developmental delays, jerky body movements, poor coordination, or nystagmus (see **Darting Eyes,** above).

There's no specific treatment, but sleep and rest can help. Fatigue and illness, on the other hand, can set off subsequent episodes. The good news is that in most cases, PTU spontaneously disappears by the time a child is 4 years of age.

DOWNCAST EYES

Q: Our 4-month-old often looks like he's gazing downward even when there's nothing there. What can this mean?

A: A downward gaze—sometimes referred to as *hypotropia*—is another form of *strabismus*. Like hypertropia, it can be a sign of *Duane syndrome* (see **An Up-Cast Eye,** above). When it is persistent, though, it can also be an important warning sign of a serious but rare condition called *setting-sun phenomenon*. With this condition, the lower part of the eyes may also be covered by the lower eyelid. Setting-sun syndrome is believed to be the result of intracranial pressure and is often an earlier sign of *hydrocephalus* than an enlarged head (see Chapter 1).

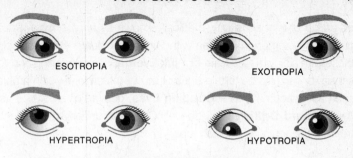

ESOTROPIA

EXOTROPIA

HYPERTROPIA

HYPOTROPIA

DIFFERENT TYPES OF STRABISMUS

Any child with this sign should be immediately evaluated by a pediatric neurologist. There is a benign form of this disorder (called *benign setting-sun phenomenon*), which is sometimes seen in babies younger than 7 months. However, if the child does have setting-sun syndrome, immediate surgery is required to prevent brain damage.

EYE-RELATED BEHAVIOR

SQUINTING

Q: *I'm a nanny for an infant who squints a lot. Can young babies be nearsighted?*

A: Squinting is, in fact, a common sign of nearsightedness at all ages, and is medically known as *myopia*. Myopic children can't see distant objects clearly and usually need eyeglasses or contact lenses to correct their nearsightedness.

Your charge's squinting may also

be a sign of light sensitivity, medically known as *photophobia*. Photophobia is common in children with very light-colored eyes, especially those with albinism (see **Pale or Pink Eyes,** above). Squinting and light sensitivity can also be telltale signs of an eye infection, a vision problem such as glaucoma (see **Protruding Eyes,** above), or amblyopia (see **An Outward-Drifting Eye,** above). Once the underlying problem is treated, the squinting should stop.

BLINKING AND WINKING

Q: Our toddler has recently started blinking a lot. Might she have an eye problem?

A: Frequent blinking is seen quite often in young children. In most cases, it's a habit or facial tic and not related to any physical disorder. More boys than girls are apt to acquire this rather disturbing (to the parents) habit, which tends to get worse when a child is tired, anxious, or bored. The good news is that most children will outgrow it in a few months.

Excessive blinking can also be a warning sign that something is irritating the child's eye, such as an eyelash, a speck of dirt, or some other tiny foreign object. Even if only one eye is affected, the child may blink both eyes. Once the offending object is removed the blinking usually stops.

A variety of eye and vision disorders can also cause a child to blink a lot. These include eye allergies and infections, vision problems, light sensitivity, and esotropia (see **Crossed Eyes,** above). In rare cases, frequent blinking can be a sign of a neurological condition such as epilepsy. If the underlying cause of these conditions can be treated successfully, the excessive blinking will usually subside.

SIGNIFICANT FACTS

- Infants blink only 1 or 2 times per minute.
- The frequency of blinking increases steadily until adolescence.
- Adolescents blink about 10 to 12 times per minute.
- The average adult blinks up to 15 times per minute, with about 1 blink every 4 seconds.
- We tend to blink more when we talk and less when we read.

If there's no apparent cause, excessive blinking can signal *blepharospasm,* aka *benign essential blepharospasm* (*BEB*). (Unfortunately, the term *blepharospasm* is sometimes mistakenly used as an umbrella term for excessive blinking, regardless of the cause.) BEB is a rare movement disorder in which the eyes (usually both) involuntarily and repeatedly blink or twitch. This progressive, neurological disorder affects more girls than boys, and can range from mild to severe. In severe cases, BEB can lead to vision loss.

When children (or adults) with blepharospasm develop other involuntary facial movements, such as grimacing, lip puckering, or chin thrusting, it's known as *Meige's syndrome.* Although there is no cure for either blepharospasm or Meige's syndrome, medical and behavioral treatments can help.

If the blinking affects only one eye and resembles winking, it may actually be an eye twitch. This involuntary eyelid spasm, medically known as *lid myokymia,* is often set off by fatigue, stress, and caffeine. (Remember, caffeine is found not just in coffee but in tea, cola drinks, and chocolate as well.) Lid myokymia is usually a benign and self-limiting condition.

WARNING SIGN

 Babies born with *fetal alcohol syndrome* (*FAS*) tend to blink less frequently than other babies. This eye-blink deficit, in fact, may be the only sign of FAS. Not all babies display the typical telltale facial signs of FAS, which include small eyes, a thin upper lip, a short upturned nose, and a small head circumference.

LACK OF EYE CONTACT

Q: *My infant son seems to have difficultly making eye contact, even when he's nursing. Isn't this a sign of autism? Or could he have something else wrong with him?*

A: It takes most babies 8 to 12 weeks before they can focus clearly enough to make direct eye contact. Poor eye contact can also be a warning sign of a vision problem, which even newborns can have.

While lack of eye contact is a hallmark of autism, a child has to display a number of other key signs before a definitive diagnosis can be made. These signs include not smiling in response to someone else's smile, especially by the age of 6 months, and not pointing to themselves or objects by the age of 12 months.

Until recently, most children with autism were not diagnosed until they were 3 or 4 years old. But today, professionals are able to diagnose autism even in young babies. Indeed, the American Academy of Pediatrics recommends that all babies be screened for autism starting at 18 months and again at 24 months.

WARNING SIGNS

 Signs of autism sometimes seen in babies younger than 18 months include:

- Lack of eye contact
- Lack of facial expression
- Not smiling in response to someone else's smile, especially by age 6 months
- Not turning toward a person who says their name
- Not engaging in back-and-forth babbling
- Not pointing to themselves or objects by age 12 months

The earlier a child is diagnosed with autism, the sooner treatment can begin, and the better the prognosis. While autism is not presently curable, early intervention can reverse or control some of its serious developmental and social consequences.

SIGNING OFF

A newborn's eyes are carefully examined at birth and at every subsequent checkup. This involves evaluation of the position, shape, size, and color of a baby's eyes. Their eyes are also checked for infections, cataracts, and glaucoma. If your baby wasn't born in a hospital, be sure that his or her eyes are checked within the first few days by a pediatrician or other qualified healthcare provider.

While doctors are likely to notice most congenital eye-related problems, parents are often the ones who first notice other eye signs, both benign and serious. Virtually all eye-related signs, whether mentioned in this chapter or not, necessitate medical evaluation. Some, however, may require immediate medical attention to save a child's eyesight or even life.

NOTIFY YOUR BABY'S PEDIATRICIAN OR OTHER HEALTHCARE PROVIDER IMMEDIATELY, OR CALL 911, IF:

- Your baby suddenly seems unable to see
- Your baby suddenly has:
  - A change in pupil size
  - A drooping of the eyelid
  - A bulging of the eye
  - Bleeding from the eye
  - Severe photosensitivity

Babies with eye problems, whether minor or major, are often referred to pediatric ophthalmologists. In rare cases, a pediatric neurologist or other specialist may need to be consulted.

CHAPTER 4

YOUR BABY'S EARS

Do your ears hang low?
Do they waggle to and fro?
Can you tie them in a knot?
Can you tie them in a bow?
—Children's song

MANY PREGNANT WOMEN WILL ADMIT—even boast—that they listen to Beethoven or Bach with the hope that it will soothe their unborn babies or even enhance their children's musical ability. Indeed, babies do hear sounds before birth. But it may not be the philharmonic. More likely they'll be hearing the sounds of their mother's bodies, and only a few (if any) sounds originating outside of the womb.

After birth, moms and dads sing and talk to their babies, which is how babies learn to speak. This phenomenal event is done almost effortlessly if all the components of hearing (to say nothing of the tongue and mouth) are in place. (See Chapter 6.) Indeed, without good hearing, speech and language development is hindered.

The first things that parents notice about their newborn's ears is their shape, size, and even position. But parents are not the only ones inspecting their babies' ears; the babies' pediatricians do so as well. Where the ears are located on a baby's head and how they look both inside and out can give these doctors clues to how well a baby hears now, and how well he or she may hear in the future. A baby's ears can also display signs of benign or serious medical conditions.

EAR SHAPES

We hardly notice our ears or those of others unless they protrude or are misshapen. Fortunately, ears that protrude—sometimes called *lop* or *outstanding* ears—are usually just a cosmetic concern. Some ear deformities, however, may be associated with various medical conditions and genetic abnormalities. That's because a baby's ears and other organs—in particular the kidneys—are developing in the womb at the same time.

The structure of the outer ear is very complex. So complex, in fact, that it can be a challenge for even the most proficient reconstructive surgeons to reproduce.

> **SIGN OF THE TIMES**
>
> In the Chinese culture, some believe long ears signify nobility and predict a long life; thick earlobes are thought to predict great wealth.

DIMPLED EAR

Q: Our daughter has a little indent right in front of her ear. A friend of mine said that it isn't just a dimple—that it could be serious. Is she right?

A: Your friend may or may not be correct. Some ear "dimples" may be *preauricular pits,* small indentations that can occur on either or both

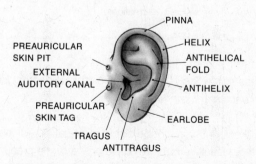

PREAURICULAR SKIN PIT · EXTERNAL AUDITORY CANAL · PREAURICULAR SKIN TAG · TRAGUS · ANTITRAGUS · PINNA · HELIX · ANTIHELICAL FOLD · ANTIHELIX · EARLOBE

OUTER EAR ANATOMY AND COMMON EAR ABNORMALITIES

ears. Preauricular pits, which are not unusual and often run in families, occur during the early stages of an embryo's development. They're seen in about 1% of white children, 5% of black children, and 10% of Asian children.

Although they're usually of no medical concern, they can become infected. The signs of an infected pit include redness and swelling. A baby may wince if the area is touched, and you may see a puslike discharge. If these infections recur frequently, surgery may be needed.

WARNING SIGN

Preauricular pits are sometimes so small that they're missed at the newborn examination. Be sure to mention any such indentation to the pediatrician at your child's next well-baby visit.

Preauricular pits can sometimes be an early sign of a very rare inherited condition called *branchio-oto-renal* (*BOR*) *syndrome* (aka *Melnick-Fraser syndrome*). People born with BOR can have neck (*branchio*) and kidney (*renal*) deformities, as well as ear (*oto*) deformities. Most children with BOR syndrome have some form of hearing loss, which can range in severity from mild to profound.

STOP SIGN

Because ear and kidney deformities commonly occur together, a renal ultrasound should be done on babies with an ear anomaly if:
- The baby's family has a history of deafness or ear or kidney deformities.
- The baby's mother had gestational diabetes.
- The baby has other physical malformations.

EAR TAG

Q: Our son has a little flap of skin in the front of his ear that looks like a skin tag. Can babies get skin tags?

A: It sounds like your son might be displaying what's medically called a *preauricular tag*. Usually a baby will have only a single preauricular tag on one ear. But sometimes one or more can appear on both ears. This fleshy knob of skin doesn't cause any discomfort and is usually nothing to worry about. However, some infants with preauricular tags or pits (see **Dimpled Ear,** above) are at increased risk of hearing impairment. Babies

SIGN OF THE TIMES

According to American folklore, baby boys who wore earrings would never grow up to be musicians.

with more obvious and serious ear and other conditions may also have these tags.

EAR BUMPS

Q: *While babysitting a neighbor's child, I noticed some bubblelike growths in front of her ear. Might this be serious?*

A: What you describe sounds like a congenital condition called *accessory auricular appendages,* which are similar to preauricular tags (see **Ear Tag,** above). These growths are actually bits of skin, fatty tissue, and sometimes cartilage. They're usually benign but may be removed for cosmetic reasons. That said, some babies born with these growths may have decreased hearing in the affected ear. Therefore, all babies with accessory auricular appendages should have frequent hearing tests.

WRINKLED EAR

Q: *My sister's son was born with one small and slightly shriveled ear. He's otherwise perfectly normal. What could have caused this?*

A: Your nephew may have *microtia,* a rare, usually benign, congenital malformation of the outer ear (*pinna*), which occurs in only 1 to 3 out of every 10,000 births. It tends to run in families and is more commonly seen in boys than in girls. In most cases, only one ear is affected, usually the right. These incomplete ear formations can range in severity from one ear being a bit smaller than the other to one being totally absent.

Interestingly, this condition is seen more often in babies born to mothers with diabetes and those born at high altitudes. Also at increased risk are babies whose mothers used alcohol or took certain drugs during pregnancy, such as isotretinoin (Accutane), which is used to treat acne, and thalidomide, which has been linked to other birth defects.

WARNING SIGN

Some babies—usually those born to diabetic mothers—are born with hairy ears (medically known as *hairy pinna*). Any baby who has hairy ears and whose mother has diabetes should be tested for thyroid disease.

Although usually a benign sign, microtia can be a warning sign of hearing loss. This type of ear malformation is sometimes seen in children with other facial deformities, usually of the lower part of the face, which would be obvious at birth. In some cases, microtia can occur with certain potentially serious medical conditions, such as kidney problems. To be safe, all babies with microtia should be thoroughly evaluated.

Depending on the severity of the problem, plastic reconstructive surgery is an option. This surgery can be quite complicated and is usually scheduled when the child is 7 years of age or older.

SIGNIFICANT FACT

Ears are among the first parts of the body to reach full size, usually at about age 5 or 6. Any corrective surgery for an ear deformity is usually delayed until then.

SIGNIFICANT FACTS

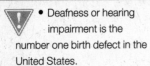

* Deafness or hearing impairment is the number one birth defect in the United States.
* About 2 to 3 out of every 1,000 children in the United States are born deaf or have a hearing deficit.
* Nine out of every 10 children who are born deaf are born to parents who can hear.

HEARING PROBLEMS

Parents may think that just because their baby becomes startled by or turns toward a loud sound, he or she couldn't possibly have a hearing problem. Unfortunately, this isn't necessarily true. Most babies who have a hearing impairment can hear some sounds. And some will react to their surroundings through their other senses, especially sight and touch. When it seems like a baby is reacting to noise, he or she may actually be reacting to a strong vibration.

Interestingly, in 2 out of 3 cases, it's the parents who are the first to suspect that something is wrong with their child's hearing. They might catch on because their baby isn't responding to loud sounds or to their voices, or because he or she is having difficulty learning to talk. The good news is that early recognition of a hearing problem can lead to effective treatment.

> **SIGN OF THE TIMES**
>
> In Italy in the Middle Ages, some "experts" believed that the way a baby responded to sound was a sign of his temperament. If an infant reacted to snapped fingers, he was best suited to masculine pursuits, especially the art of war. But if the baby showed a preference for lullabies and poetry, he was better suited to a life of study and science. It's not clear how they interpreted a baby girl's response to certain sounds.

SMALL BABIES AND HEARING

Q: Our baby was a preemie. We're thankful he's very healthy, but I've heard that premature babies often have hearing problems. Should we worry?

A: Babies who are born prematurely, as well as low-birth-weight babies (less than 3½ pounds), are indeed at increased risk for having a hearing problem. In fact, any baby—whether full-term or premature—who was in neonatal intensive care, had a respiratory problem that required breathing machines, or had a blood transfusion is at increased risk of developing hearing problems.

BORN DEAF

Q: I heard that most babies with hearing problems are born that way. Is that true?

> **SIGN OF THE TIMES**
>
> For many deaf children in the United States, American Sign Language (ASL) is their first language. This is also true for the growing number of normal-hearing babies who are part of the new baby sign language movement. Because babies only babble, they have trouble communicating their needs, which leads to frustration, and possibly temper tantrums. Proponents say sign language gives babies an easy way to "tell" their parents what's going on. They claim that it also promotes language and social skills, and self-esteem. ASL is the 4th most frequently used language in the United States.

HEARING (AND SPEECH) MILESTONES

Birth to 3 months	3 to 6 months	6 to 12 months	12 to 15 months	15 to 24 months	24 months to 36 months
Startles at a loud noise.	Quiets down when hearing your voice.	Responds to own name, a telephone ringing, a person's voice.	Responds to "no."	Points to pictures when you say the object's name.	Understands simple abstract phrases (e.g., "Not now" and "No more").
Wakes up if there's a sudden loud noise.	Stops to listen to a new sound.	Knows words for common things (e.g., bottle, shoe) and sayings (e.g.,"Bye-bye!").	Understands simple requests.	Points to some body parts when asked.	Can choose between objects if asked for by size (e.g., "big cookie").
Blinks or widens eyes when there's a sudden noise.	Looks for the source of a new sound.	Makes babbling sounds, even when alone.	Imitates sounds.	Listens to stories, songs, or rhythms.	Follows simple, 2-step commands (e.g., "Get your sweater and bring it here").
	Smiles when spoken to by parent.	Responds to requests (e.g., "Come here").	Tries to say words.	Speaks several words.	Understands many action words (e.g., run, jump).
		Looks at things or pictures when someone refers to them.			

A: Most hearing impairment in children is *congenital* (present at birth) and can be either inherited or not. But babies can develop hearing loss later on from a wide variety of causes, including injury, recurrent infection, a genetic condition, or exposure in the womb to a maternal infection.

Several types of infection acquired after birth can cause hearing problems too. For example, babies who've had meningitis, mumps, or measles, or who were exposed in the womb to certain other serious bacterial and viral infections, are at increased risk. The same is true for babies with jaundice. (See Chapter 3.)

Hearing loss can also be an inherited trait. Those children with close relatives who suffered from permanent hearing loss before age 30 are especially at risk.

SIGNIFICANT FACT

Not only can meningitis cause hearing loss, but, according to a recent Danish study, children with hearing loss are at increased risk of meningitis. Cochlear implants, which are used to treat serious hearing loss, increase the risk of meningitis. Because of this, the Centers for Disease Control (CDC) recommends that children with these implants get vaccinated against the leading causes of meningitis.

STOP SIGN

Because some disorders that cause hearing loss in children also lead to vision loss, all children with impaired hearing should have at least 1 eye examination with a pediatric ophthalmologist.

EAR INFECTIONS AND HEARING LOSS

Q: *My 8-month-old daughter had her first ear infection. I've heard so much about ear infections leading to hearing loss. Should I be concerned?*

A: It's true that ear infections, which are very common in babies, can lead to hearing loss. But not all children who get ear infections—even repeated ones—develop hearing loss. Ironically,

SIGNIFICANT FACTS

- By their 1st birthday, 60% to 80% of infants will have had at least 1 ear infection.
- By age 5, 75% to 95% of children will experience at least 1 ear infection.
- Between 20% and 25% of children will get more than 6 ear infections.

SIGN OF THE TIMES

Here are some old American folk remedies for earaches:

- Put cockroach juice in the ear.
- Make eardrops out of the broth of goose manure.
- Rub the ear with rabbit urine.

a recent hearing problem may be a warning sign of an ear infection.

The signs of ear infection, medically called *otitis media,* can be subtle or come in loud and clear. It's important to be attuned to these signs, which often appear suddenly. In infants and toddlers, behavioral signs may include fussiness, inconsolable crying, rubbing or pulling of the ears, difficulty falling asleep, and not eating. Toddlers may also have trouble keeping their balance when they walk.

A yellowish or reddish discharge from the ear, or even from the eye, can also signal an ear infection. (Of course, fever is a common sign too, occurring in about half of children younger than 3 years of age who have an ear infection.) Some parents will notice other signs such as hearing loss, which is caused by a buildup of fluid in the middle ear. This will usually resolve after treatment, which typically involves antibiotics.

STOP SIGN

Here are some tips that may help reduce your baby's risk of ear infection:

- Try to limit your baby's time in day care, where germs can be passed around.
- Keep your baby away from cigarette smoke.
- Breast-feed as long as possible.
- Ask your baby's pediatrician about the pneumococcal vaccine. (The American Academy of Pediatrics recommends this vaccination for all children younger than 2 years of age.)

The good news is that there are several measures now available to help prevent recurrent ear infections and hearing impairment.

WARNING SIGN

In a test of more than 200 noise-producing toys, only 10 fell within acceptable noise levels set by the U.S. Occupational Safety and Health Administration. All the others could place children at risk for hearing damage.

EAR- AND HEARING-RELATED BEHAVIORS

STUFFING STUFF IN THE EARS

Q: *My 2-year-old son has been putting things in his ears. Why does he do it?*

A: Young children often put objects in their ears, as well as in their noses and mouths. (See Chapter 5 and Chapter 6.) Sometimes it's a sign of boredom, sometimes exploration. Also, some children who have chronic outer ear infections will put things in their ears to try to relieve discomfort. Whatever the reason, inserting foreign bodies in the ear can be more than just a momentary irritation for parents.

Both boys and girls are equally likely to place things in their ears—as well as those of siblings and playmates. High on the favorites list are toy parts, eraser tips, crayon pieces, hair beads, wads of paper, and food. Button batteries (the small batteries that power watches and some electronic toys) in the ear are a particularly important medical emergency. They can very quickly leak corrosive materials that can damage the ears.

Sometimes the only signs that a child has put something in his or her ear are rubbing or pulling on the ear. Drainage or redness are other common signs of an unsuspected foreign object in the ear.

If an object gets stuck in a baby's ear, it can lead to inflammation, infection, a perforated eardrum, or even hearing loss. In fact, recent hearing loss may be the first sign that a child has stuck something in his or her ear. While some foreign objects dislodge

SPEAKING OF SIGNS

Why did the kids put beans in their ears?
No one can hear with beans in their ears.
After a while the reason appears.
They did it 'cause we said no.

—From the Harvey Schmidt and Tom Jones musical *The Fantasticks,* 1960

SIGN OF THE TIMES

People who can move and wiggle their ears at will have been born with highly developed auricular muscles. This "anomaly"—or trick, as some might say—was mentioned by the 4th-century theologian and philosopher St. Augustine in his writings.

on their own, others, such as food and batteries, are more difficult—and dangerous—and should be removed by a healthcare professional.

STOP SIGN

(STOP) Don't try to remove a foreign object from your child's ear. It can get lodged deeper in the ear. And the object—or what you use to remove it—can damage the ear's delicate tissues.

DEAFNESS OR AUTISM?

Q: I've heard that some children are mistakenly thought to have hearing problems when, in fact, they are tuning out because they're autistic. How can you tell the difference?

A: Indeed, some parents of children with autism may initially think that their child has a hearing problem. Autism is a complex developmental disability that affects the ability to communicate, interact, or connect with others in a meaningful way. (See Chapter 3.) But it takes skilled professionals to make a definitive diagnosis. There are some hearing-related signs, however, that help point to whether a child is hearing-impaired or autistic.

SIGN OF THE TIMES

The American Academy of Pediatrics now urges all children to be screened for autism at 18 months and 24 months, even if there's no reason to suspect the disorder. Early recognition and intervention can help improve the lives of children with autism.

Autistic children tend to react to sounds and other sensory stimuli differently than other children. For example, some autistic children have selective hearing—they'll hear and "connect" with environmental sounds, but not human voices. And some act as if they don't hear anything. On the other hand, others are highly sensitive to sounds; they may jump at sudden noises or cover their ears.

One of the earliest signs of autism in babies—one that's easily confused with hearing loss—is their inability to respond to their names. Children normally react to their names at a very early age, usually by 8 to 10 months. Autistic children don't. Of course, children with hearing impairments may not either, but they may turn their heads when called because they can see you or can tell you're there. (See Chapter 3.)

Autism, or more accurately *autism spectrum disorders* (ASD), covers a wide range of behaviors and abilities. Not all autistic children display the same signs or act the same. If you think your child is acting in an unusual way, you should consult his or her pediatrician.

SIGNING OFF

A newborn's ears are part of the routine neonatal examination in a hospital. The location, size, and appearance of the infant's ears, both inside and out, will be evaluated. And the baby's inner and outer ear will be checked again at each subsequent well-baby visit.

In 37 states (and Washington, D.C.), universal hearing screening is required before a newborn leaves a hospital or birthing center. Most other states recommend screening of all newborns before 1 month of age. If you think your baby wasn't screened in the hospital or birthing center, or if he or she was born at home, make sure his or her hearing is checked within the first month of life. If needed, a baby will undergo further testing and intervention before 3 months of age; children at high risk for hearing loss should then be screened every 6 months until they are 3 years of age.

Parents are often the first to observe hearing problems in their children after the newborn period and should report their concerns to the pediatrician as soon as possible. In addition, there are certain ear-related signs that require immediate medical attention.

NOTIFY YOUR CHILD'S HEALTHCARE PROVIDER IMMEDIATELY IF YOUR BABY:

- Suddenly seems to have lost hearing
- Has something stuck in the ear
- Has sustained a serious injury or blow to the ear
- Has a bloody discharge or clear fluid coming from the ear

A pediatrician can diagnose and treat many common and uncommon ear conditions. However, some ear-related disorders may require help from ear, nose, and throat (ENT) specialists, allergists, neurologists, audiologists, speech therapists, or other healthcare professionals.

CHAPTER 5

YOUR BABY'S NOSE

Ring around the rosy.
Pocket full of posies.
Achoo! Achoo!
We all fall down.
—Popular British nursery rhyme

A BABY'S NOSE IS ONE of his or her most noteworthy appendages. For one thing, newborns breathe through their noses, not their mouths. And it's through their noses, rather than their eyes, that infants first recognize their mothers. Indeed, at birth, they're able to identify the smell of their mother's milk, which helps them home in on her nipples.

Fetuses get their first sniff of their moms while they're still in the womb. In fact, scientists recently discovered that 27-week-old fetuses can sense the estimated 120 different scents found in amniotic fluid. Although they don't breathe in the normal sense, fetuses take amniotic fluid into their lungs through their noses. At birth, an infant's lungs are still filled with fluid, and bubbles

SIGNIFICANT FACTS

- At birth, a baby's sense of smell is about 10,000 times more accurate than his or her sense of taste.
- Newborns can even recognize their mothers by their odor.

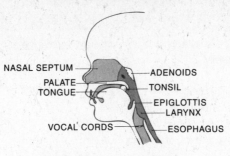

NASAL SEPTUM
PALATE
TONGUE
VOCAL CORDS
ADENOIDS
TONSIL
EPIGLOTTIS
LARYNX
ESOPHAGUS

NOSE AND THROAT ANATOMY

may come out of his or her nose. Newborns also tend to sneeze a lot, which helps clear their noses.

Many parents are dismayed to find that their baby is born with a squished or swollen nose. Pressure on the face during the ride out of the birth canal is usually to blame. The good news is that by the end of the first week, most newborns will have a normal-looking nose.

As the infant grows, so does his or her nose, in significance as well as size. For example, the sense of smell becomes extremely important when a baby starts eating solid food.

The nose can also be a wellspring of clues about a baby's health. By paying attention to nasal shapes, sounds, and secretions, parents can learn to sniff out problems before they become too serious.

> **SIGNIFICANT FACT**
>
> A mother does not even have to be present for her scent to affect her baby. Researchers have found that a piece of cloth that a mother had previously draped over her shoulder can help soothe a fussy baby when placed in the baby's crib.

FLARING NOSTRILS

Q: When our infant daughter breathes, her nostrils widen. Is this normal?

A: Nasal flaring is not only normal but actually necessary for newborns; it helps infants breathe when breast-feeding. However, when a baby is not nursing and his or her nostrils persistently flare, it can signal a breathing problem. This can result from any number of conditions, including nasal or airway obstruction, asthma, croup, or pneumonia.

HAIRLESS BUMP ON
THE NOSE

Q: *My toddler has a lump over the tip of her nose. It doesn't seem to
bother her, but it bothers me. Should I be concerned?*

A: A bump on the nose can be any number of things ranging from a
pimple to a tumor. But if your child was born with the bump, it could be
a very rare, benign growth called a *nasal glioma*. (Nasal gliomas are not
cancerous and should not be confused with brain gliomas, which can
be malignant.) These growths are more common in boys than in girls.

Nasal gliomas are usually firm but not tender to the touch. They can
be red or blue, which can make them look like hemangiomas, a common birthmark. (See Chapter 8.) Although sometimes found inside the
nose, most are on the outside. Ones that start on the outside, though,
can occasionally spread inside. Whether initially small or large, nasal
gliomas can grow, possibly blocking a nostril and making breathing difficult. Sometimes children with these growths will snore. (See **Small
Snorers,** below.) In rare cases, nasal gliomas can grow so large that
the bridge of the baby's nose becomes deformed.

Unlike *nasal dermoid cysts* (see **Hairy Bump on the Nose,** below),
nasal gliomas don't have hair growing out of them, nor do they usually
ooze. But some of these nasal growths actually have a connection with
parts of the skull, which can cause *cerebrospinal fluid,* the very clear,
watery liquid that's in and around the brain and spinal cord, to leak out
of the nostrils. This may be a sign that the glioma is burrowed deeper
into the back of the nose toward the skull, a condition that raises the
risk of meningitis. Tearing from the eye is also fairly common in children

with these growths. Surgery is usually needed to prevent recurrence and nose and facial deformities.

HAIRY BUMP ON THE NOSE

Q: I heard that a small hairy lump on a baby's nose can be a sign of a serious problem. Is that true?

A: A bump on the nose that has hair growing from it is the hallmark of a *nasal dermoid cyst*. This is a rare, congenital condition that's more common in boys than in girls. Sometimes these cysts are so small they're not even noticed until they cause problems. They are sometimes seen in babies who have other more obvious anomalies, such as a cleft palate.

Dermoid cysts, which can occur on various other parts of the body besides the nose, contain hair follicles and *sebaceous* (oil) glands. They're often flesh-colored or yellow. Some nasal dermoid cysts go deep under the skin, with potentially serious consequences—they can become inflamed and infected, and can ooze pus or fatty material. Because nasal dermoid cysts are so close to the brain and skull, they can cause a brain abscess and can lead to infection and even deformity of the skull bones. They can also lead to meningitis. Surgery is usually necessary to remove these growths and prevent damage to the nose, face, and skull.

NASAL CREASE

Q: I've recently noticed that my 2-year-old son has a long crease over his nose. What could cause this?

A: A long crinkle over the nose is often a sign of a nasal allergy. Children (and adults) with such allergies, particularly those with chronic allergies, will often try to relieve their unrelentingly itchy or drippy noses by rubbing them repeatedly with the palms of their hands in an upward motion. This repetitive motion is medically referred to as the *nasal salute*. When the allergy is treated, the nasal crease should gradually disappear.

RUNNY NOSE

Q: How do I know whether my baby's runny nose is a cold or an allergy?

A: That's a question that often perplexes physicians as well as parents. Though there are no hard-and-fast rules, here are some basic guidelines

SIGNIFICANT FACTS

Here are some facts about colds:

- Mothers pass along temporary immunity to cold viruses to their newborns—but only to those that they themselves have been exposed to. At about 6 months of age, this immunity wears off and children become susceptible to the more than 200 existing cold viruses. From then on, babies and children can develop immunity to cold viruses, but only one at a time.
- Two-year-olds in day care get about twice as many colds as those cared for at home. But between ages 6 and 11, they have ⅓ fewer colds than those who were stay-at-home babies do.
- The average child has about 6 to 10 colds a year.
- Children who have siblings in school get an average of 12 colds a year.

that will help you detect the source of your child's runny nose.

A child with a cold may sneeze once or twice, but a child with an allergy will sneeze rapidly and repeatedly. And in children with nasal allergies, there's usually a pattern to when the sneezing or nasal discharge starts—for example, you may notice that it happens most often in the spring or when the child is around a cat.

While nasal allergies are usually caused by environmental or other irritants, the common cold, medically known as an *upper respiratory tract infection,* can be caused by any of more than 200 viruses. In both a cold and an allergy, the nasal discharge is thin and watery, but the nasal discharge from a cold often becomes thicker—and possibly yellowish (a day or two after the runny nose starts)—before the cold runs its course.

However, yellow or greenish nasal mucus that persists for longer than a week is more often a sign of a bacterial infection in the nose, sinuses, or throat than of a cold. This type of infection usually requires antibiotics, whereas a cold doesn't. Indeed, antibiotics aren't effective against viral infections.

WARNING SIGN

In 2008, the Food and Drug Administration (FDA) issued a public health advisory that over-the-counter (OTC) cough and cold products should not be given to infants and children under 2 years of age because serious and potentially life-threatening side effects could develop.

DANGEROUS COLDS

Q: *My mother says some colds in babies can be so serious that they require hospitalization. Is she right?*

A: Yes, your mother is correct. Some colds are caused by a common, highly contagious, and potentially dangerous virus called *respiratory syncytial virus (RSV)*. Although almost all children are infected with RSV by their 2nd birthday without any serious consequences, a small percentage will develop complications and require hospitalization. RSV is the most common cause of *bronchiolitis* (inflammation of the small airways in the lung) and *pneumonia* in children younger than 1 year of age in the United States. In fact, 75,000 to 125,000 children in this age group are hospitalized due to RSV annually in the United States each year.

> **STOP SIGN**
>
> **STOP** The Centers for Disease Control (CDC) recommends that people with colds should avoid contact with children at high risk for respiratory syncytial virus (RSV). Here are some other precautions that you or anyone with a cold should follow to help prevent the spread of RSV and other viruses.
> - Cover your coughs and sneezes.
> - Wash your hands frequently and correctly (with soap and water for 15 to 20 seconds).
> - Don't share cups and eating utensils.
> - Refrain from kissing others.
> - Clean contaminated surfaces (such as doorknobs and toys).

RSV tends to occur less often in the summer than in the other seasons. Children may have repeated bouts of it. The signs of RSV are similar to those of the common cold: stuffy or runny nose, cough, wheezing, fever, and loss of appetite. It usually takes 1 to 2 weeks for an RSV infection to run its course. Children with the more serious RSV infections will usually have thick yellow or green nasal discharge and a high fever. They may also have breathing difficulty and a worsening cough that produces yellow, green, or gray phlegm.

RSV is most serious in the very young—particularly babies under 6 months of age. Premature babies and those with underlying problems such as heart, lung, and immunological conditions are at particular risk for RSV complications. Children who wheeze are also more likely to have serious RSV infections.

In most cases, RSV should be treated like any other cold. Because it's a virus, antibiotics are of no help unless a bacterial infection is also present. In more serious cases, however, a child usually requires intravenous fluids and other treatments that are available only in the hospital.

SUN SNEEZING

Q: *Our baby girl sneezes whenever I take her outside. I don't think it's an allergy because she stops after a few sneezes. What else might be causing this?*

SIGN OF THE TIMES

Ancient Egyptians thought that looking at the sun and sneezing would bring good luck.

A: It sounds like your baby has a very common condition known as *photic sneezing*. Up to 1 in 3 people sneeze when they go out in the sun! It's thought to be a hereditary trait and those of European descent are more predisposed to it than those of Asian or African descent.

Photic sneezing is known by many other names, including *solar sneeze reflex, light sneeze reflex,* and last but not least the *ACHOO syndrome,* which stands for *autosomal dominant compelling helio-ophthalmic outburst syndrome.* Whatever it's called, it's not only quite common but totally harmless.

SIGN OF THE TIMES

Aristotle believed that the heat of the sun on the nose was the cause of sun sneezing. Two millennia later, Sir Francis Bacon disproved this theory by going out in the sun with his eyes closed. No sneeze ensued. He reasoned: The sun caused the eyes to produce tears, which then seeped into the nose, causing nasal irritation and sneezes.

BABY BREATHS

SMALL SNORERS

Q: *Our baby boy snores. Why is this and does it mean that he'll be just like his dad and always snore?*

A: Snoring is common in infants and babies, particularly boys. Because a baby's nasal passages are quite narrow, it's not unusual for them to fill up with secretions. When air passes through these secretions during sleep, it causes a vibration or snorelike sound. Toddlers—particularly those older than 3 years—tend to snore during the deep stages of sleep. This typical type of snoring, called *primary snoring,* is not

associated with any serious medical problem, and many will outgrow this. When a child continues to snore habitually with no obvious cause, though, it may be a sign of some structural problem with his or her nasal passages.

Snoring is also fairly common in children with colds or allergies. When the cold or allergy is gone, the nocturnal noise will most likely go away too.

Snoring in children can occasionally be a warning sign of a sleep-related breathing problem, medically known as *obstructive sleep apnea* (OSA). OSA can be caused by enlarged tonsils and adenoids. Other possible causes include obesity and acid reflux, aka GERD. (See **Breathing Breaks,** below.) GERD, which stands for *gastrointestinal reflux disease,* is a common condition in babies and is believed to cause spitting up and colic. Once these problems resolve, the OSA and snoring tend to improve.

Children with facial or head abnormalities also tend to snore. Finally, there is a genetic component: Infants who snore are likely to have parents who snore. Usually these nose noises stop when the baby is a little bit older, although snoring sometimes does continue throughout childhood and adulthood.

BREATHING BREAKS

Q: When our 6-month-old son sleeps, he occasionally stops breathing for a few seconds, then goes back to breathing normally. We worry, especially about SIDS. Should we?

A: All babies occasionally stop breathing for a few seconds during sleep. Often referred to as *apnea,* these short pauses—no more than about 15 seconds—are very common. Ironically, some doctors refer to these benign breathing breaks as *periodic breathing.* Premature babies and those who move around a great deal during sleep often experience these repeated interruptions in breathing.

Stopping and starting breathing many times during the night can also be a sign of *obstructive sleep apnea* (*OSA*). (See **Small Snorers,** above.) Although many babies with sleep apnea snore, sleep apnea and snoring don't always go hand in hand. Just because a baby doesn't snore doesn't mean that he or she doesn't have sleep apnea. OSA can also be a sign that a baby has an infection, or an airway obstruction, is choking, or even has a heart disorder. Here's the good news: If there's no medical cause for the sleep apnea, the baby will likely outgrow it.

There's another type of apnea that's more serious, called *ALTE,* which stands for *apparent life-threatening event.* This involves sudden, longer, more frightening episodes of apnea during which a baby may also change color, become limp, or appear to be choking or gagging.

ALTE is more common in certain babies: those younger than 12 months, boys, and those who feed rapidly, cough frequently, or appear to choke when eating. Premature babies are also more susceptible to ALTE than full-term ones, and those who've had *respiratory syncytial virus* (*RSV*) infections (see **Dangerous Colds,** above) or have undergone general anesthesia are at increased risk as well.

ALTE can signal a number of medical problems, including *gastrointestinal reflux disease* (*GERD*) (see **Small Snorers,** above), an irregular

DANGER SIGN

 If your baby appears to stop breathing for 20 seconds or longer, call 911 or take him or her to the emergency room. This may be a sign of an ALTE.

In the meantime:

- Try mild stimulation—like a flick of the fingers on the baby's feet.
- If that doesn't work, try a stronger pinch.
- If there's still no response, immediately start mouth-to-nose resuscitation.

Never shake the baby—it can cause head injury or even death!

heartbeat (*arrhythmia*), or a seizure disorder. Whether there is an association between ALTEs and *sudden infant death syndrome* (*SIDS*) is unclear. Fortunately, ALTE tends to occur less frequently as babies reach their 1st birthday.

WEE WHISTLES

Q: *My baby daughter makes a whistling sound when she breathes. Should we worry?*

A: Infants can sometimes produce a high-pitched, musical, or whistle-like sound when they breathe in. Medically known as *stridor,* this can be caused by a bit of mucus or even dried milk blocking their small nasal passages, which can make it hard for little babies to move air in and out of their noses.

Stridor can also signal some potentially serious respiratory problems, including nasal allergies, infections, and injury. Babies with throat, larynx (*voice box*) (see Chapter 6), or trachea (*windpipe*) malformations may also have stridor. When the underlying cause is treated, the stridor usually stops.

In an older baby, a whistling sound may be a red flag that something's been shoved into the nose and may have become lodged in the lung or esophagus. (See **Shoving Stuff up the Nose,** below.)

FAST OR SLOW BREATHING

Q: *I often babysit for my grandchildren. My daughter's newborn usually breathes very quickly, while her toddler breathes more slowly. Why is that?*

A: Newborns breathe about 40 times per minute, while infants take between 20 and 40 breaths each minute. (Breathing continues to slow down until adulthood; adults take an average of 12 to 20 breaths per minute.)

Babies tend to breathe faster when they're very active, upset, or crying, and they breathe differently at different times of the day and night. For example, babies often breathe more slowly when sleeping, and they may even pause for a few seconds between breaths. (See **Breathing Breaks,** above.)

Each baby has his or her own pattern of breathing, and any unusual change may signal a problem. For example, in babies younger than 6 months, fast breathing may be the only sign of an infection in the lower respiratory tract, where the small airways of the lungs are located.

Continuous rapid breathing (known as *tachypnea*) could be a sign of lung disease—in particular, pneumonia or heart problems. (This shouldn't be confused with *transient tachypnea in newborns* [*TTN*], which is a very common, benign occurrence seen in babies younger than 2 days old and usually resolves itself within a day or two.) On the other hand, very long pauses between breaths (apnea) may be a warning of several potentially serious conditions. (See **Breathing Breaks,** above.)

NOSE-RELATED BEHAVIOR

SHOVING STUFF UP THE NOSE

Q: *Our toddler sometimes sticks cotton or pieces of tissue into her nose. Why would she do such a thing, and can it cause problems?*

A: It's not uncommon for young children to put odd objects into their nostrils. And noses aren't the only common destination for foreign bodies; children sometimes stick things in their ears as well. (See Chapter 4.) Besides soft items such as cotton balls and tissue paper, harder items including beads, buttons, batteries, marbles, pebbles, pieces of food, nuts, and toy parts have also wound up in the nose.

Children don't usually start putting things in their noses until about 9 months of age, when they have the coordination to hold small objects

DANGER SIGN

Button batteries are extremely dangerous if a baby puts them in his or her ear, nose, or mouth. They very quickly leak corrosive material, which can cause severe burns, sores, and facial nerve paralysis. This is a medical emergency. If not removed within an hour, these batteries can cause permanent damage to the baby.

in their fingers. They may practice this peculiar ritual out of curiosity, boredom, or copycat behavior, and may not stop doing it until they're much older. Interestingly, girls are more likely than boys to put things in their noses.

While this is usually just a harmless habit, an object can get lodged in the nose and cause problems. In that event, the child's breathing may suddenly become strained or even noisy. But this change in breathing is not always obvious, and the only discernible sign may be mucus discharge from one nostril that may be bloody or foul-smelling. Indeed, some parents go to the pediatrician's office complaining that their child "smells bad," only to find out that there's something stuck in the child's nose. The dripping may also irritate the skin around the nostril, making it red and raw.

The offending object can also cause infections anywhere along the nasal passage, especially in the sinuses. Small batteries and other objects that contain chemicals can leak into the body, causing burns. If the foreign object is pushed back far enough, it can lodge in the throat and cause vomiting, difficulty talking or breathing, or choking. Safely extracting the foreign body can be tricky, so unless the object comes out by itself, its removal is best left to a healthcare professional.

STOP SIGN

STOP If your baby has a foreign object in his or her nose:

- Don't try to get it out if it's not visible or easy to grab. You might accidentally push it farther up the nose.
- Don't ever use instruments such as tweezers or cotton swabs to remove an object. They too can push it farther up your child's nose. They can also damage the tender linings of the nose, and even perforate the part that separates the two nostrils.
- Don't try getting your child to sneeze by putting pepper under his or her nose. That can raise the risk that the object will be inhaled.

NOSE PICKING

Q: *My 2-year-old frequently picks his nose. Why is that and can it be harmful?*

A: Your toddler is not alone. It's natural for babies to explore all parts of their bodies, and the face is a convenient place to start. When they find a hole, they're likely to probe it, and tiny fingers are the perfect utensils. As babies grow older, they'll likely pick their noses for other purposes: to remove dried mucus or to scratch an itch. Children with allergies and those who live in overly dry heated or air-conditioned homes are more likely to pick up the nose-picking habit.

When nose picking becomes a habit, it's medically referred to as *rhinotillexomania*. It can be an unsightly sign of boredom or nervousness. Older children, however, may consciously pick it up to gross out their friends, their parents, or even their parents' friends!

SIGN OF THE TIMES

Archeologists have dug out evidence that cave dwellers picked their noses. And in 1350 B.C., King Tutankhamen had his own personal nose picker.

Although annoying, this habit is usually quite benign, but children who aggressively or habitually pick their noses may wind up with frequent nosebleeds, colds, and possibly serious nasal infections. In fact, vigorous nose picking can push germs and bacteria deep into the nasal cavities, causing what's called a *retrograde infection*—a potentially serious infection that can spread to other parts of the body, including the brain.

Nose picking is embarrassing enough, but much to the horror of some parents, their children may also eat their pickings. When nose picking becomes too frequent, forceful, or socially inappropriate, it's best to discuss it with your child's pediatrician, or a pediatric psychologist.

SIGN OF THE TIMES

Dr. Friedrich Bischinger, a lung specialist in Austria, believes that picking your nose and eating it is good for you. He cites 2 reasons: (1) a finger is far more effective in keeping your nose clean than a tissue and (2) eating the pickings "is a great way of strengthening your body's immune system," he argues. "The nose is a filter in which a great deal of bacteria is collected, and when this mixture arrives in the intestines it works just like a medicine."

SIGNING OFF

At birth and subsequent well-baby examinations, a baby's nose and breathing will be carefully checked. Once the baby goes home, his or her parents are likely to be the ones to notice the first signs of nasal issues, especially breathing problems. Some signs can wait until the baby's next checkup, but some should be brought to the immediate attention of the doctor, or might even require a trip to the emergency room.

NOTIFY YOUR BABY'S PEDIATRICIAN OR HEALTHCARE PROVIDER AS SOON AS POSSIBLE IF YOUR BABY:

- Has recurrent nosebleeds
- Becomes short of breath periodically, particularly when not active
- Produces a high-pitched sound (stridor) when breathing in
- Produces a wheezing sound when breathing out
- Breathes rapidly while snoring
- Wakes up frequently from snoring

GO TO THE EMERGENCY ROOM OR CALL 911 IF YOUR BABY:

- Has a nosebleed that doesn't stop within 5 to 10 minutes
- Has a button battery or other foreign object stuck in the nose
- Has had a serious injury to the nose
- Has clear, watery discharge streaming from the nose, especially after a head injury or with a fever
- Is having difficulty breathing and:
  - Turns blue (*cyanosis*)
  - Has a high fever
  - Is listless
  - Starts wheezing for the first time
  - Has a chest that looks sunken

While your baby's pediatrician can diagnose and manage many nose or breathing disorders, specialists may be needed to evaluate and treat some of them. These include ear, nose, and throat (ENT) doctors (aka *otorhinolaryngologists*), allergists, respiratory therapists, and sometimes surgeons.

CHAPTER 6

YOUR BABY'S MOUTH

Through the house what busy joy
Just because the infant boy
Has a tiny tooth to show!
—Charles and Mary Lamb,
Poetry for Children, 1809

A BABY'S MOUTH IS A marvel. Surrounded by lips, the mouth is home to the tongue, gums, and eventually the teeth. Each of these components contributes to the all-important functions of eating, tasting, and talking.

Babies' mouths have more nerve endings per square inch than any other part of their bodies. This might explain why they often explore the world with their mouths by mouthing, gumming, licking, tasting, and biting anything that fits in.

Parents may find it instructive to explore their baby's mouth as well, and pediatricians will certainly do so at birth and at each well-baby visit. Indeed, a baby's lips, tongue, gums, breath, teeth, and voice can speak volumes about his or her state of health or illness.

A BABY'S LIPS

A baby's lips are indispensable for sucking milk from a mother's breast or a bottle's nipple. The lips are not only the most visible part of the mouth but also the most appealing; they bestow smiles and kisses on their doting parents.

But lips can also tell parents when something is amiss, even if the baby can't. It's not just pouting and quivering lips that parents need to pay attention to; changes in lip color or texture can also indicate that something may be wrong.

BLUE LIPS

Q: *Our baby boy often has blue lips, even when it's warm inside. Could he possibly have some sort of heart or lung condition?*

A: Blue or even purplish lips (as well as skin, tongue, and gums) signal that the body isn't getting enough oxygen. As scary as it sounds, this condition—referred to as *cyanosis*—can be a perfectly normal occurrence. For example, when children get overly excited or have temper tantrums, their lips and mouths may turn blue, a form of cyanosis called *central cyanosis*. These spells are similar to breath holding, which is common in some children. In these benign cases, the child's tongue will remain pink and the skin color will go back to normal once the baby quiets down.

Another example of a benign cyanosis is when a chilled child's hands and feet turn bluish. This is a common condition called *peripheral cyanosis* (see Chapter 8). Once the baby warms up, the blue color will disappear.

If cyanosis persists even when a baby is resting or isn't sick, it can be a sign of a serious disorder. Blue lips can signal asthma in a child who coughs or has trouble breathing. And blue lips, skin, fingers, and fingernails can signal congenital heart defects (aka *blue baby*) or serious respiratory problems in newborns or even in older babies. Depending on the severity of the child's cardiac condition, either medication or surgery is usually needed.

BABY BLISTERS

Q: My newborn grandson has what looks like a big blister on his lip. His mother says it's from nursing, but I think his pacifier is to blame. Who's right?

A: You both may be right. Many babies younger than 6 months develop what's aptly called *sucking* or *nursing blisters*. These result from vigorous sucking, whether on their mothers' nipples, rubber nipples, or pacifiers. The blisters sometimes pop up inside a baby's mouth as well. Besides having blisters, the baby may also have slightly swollen lips. The swelling and blisters usually disappear on their own.

SIGNIFICANT FACT

Some babies are born with sucking blisters on their arms, hands, fingers, and legs from vigorously sucking on these body parts in the womb. After these babies are born, they often continue to favor these special sucking spots, if they can still reach them.

Q: Our baby's just started teething and has developed a bump on his lower lip. Can these conditions be related?

A: A lip bump can be caused by any number of things, from a bang on the lip to a bug bite. If the bump is smooth and soft, it may be a *mucocele,* a harmless, mucus-filled, cystlike swelling. Some of these mucoceles also have a bluish tint. While usually seen on the lip, they can occur inside the cheek, on the tongue, and on the roof of the mouth. They're found more frequently in girls than in boys and are usually caused by some injury, such as lip biting. The good news is that mucoceles often swell and rupture on their own without any problem. If they don't burst, they may have to be removed.

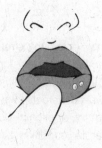

MUCOCELE

A BABY'S TONGUE

A baby's tongue serves many purposes, from helping the baby suck to helping him or her swallow milk and other liquids. As the baby grows, the tongue takes on new tasks such as sloshing solids around the mouth toward the teeth. And neither the liquids nor the solids are likely to tantalize a tot without the help of the tongue's taste buds. Finally, the tongue plays a key role in talking, singing, and even whistling. Many toddlers soon discover other uses for their tongues: blowing "raspberries" and sticking them out at rivals on the playground.

> **SIGNS OF THE TIMES**
>
> Children—and adults—in cultures throughout the world stick out their tongues. It's a friendly gesture in some Himalayan countries but an insult in European countries. For Chinese children, it signals mock terror.

The tongue is covered with microscopic hairs called *filiform papillae,* which contain the taste buds. Like the hairs on our heads, they continuously grow and shed. Those on the back of the tongue shed more slowly than those in the front and tend to be longer, making them more susceptible to bacterial and yeast infections. In fact, the tongue can have quite a taste for trouble.

> **SIGNIFICANT FACT**
>
> Every child—and adult— has a unique tongue print.

BLACKISH TONGUE

Q: *Our child's tongue has recently turned black. What could have caused this?*

A: If your child's normally pink tongue turns black—and he hasn't been licking a lot of licorice lollipops or sucking grape sour balls—it may be a sign of a condition aptly named *black hairy tongue* (aka *lingua villosa nigra*). When the tongue hairs don't shed (see **A Baby's Tongue,** above), they can overgrow and trap bacteria and food, turning the tongue dark yellow, green, brown, or even black. A black hairy tongue is also a common reaction to certain antibiotics and bismuth-containing stomach medications, such as Pepto-Bismol.

In an older child, black hairy tongue can be a telltale sign of poor oral hygiene. Regularly scraping or brushing the tongue, as well as the teeth, should help. Ironically, excessive use of mouthwash can actually cause black hairy tongue. Because mouthwash kills bacteria, its frequent use can lead to overgrowth of fungi and color-changing bacteria.

A GROOVY TONGUE

Q: Our 2-year-old daughter's tongue has deep grooves running up and down it. What could this mean?

A: It sounds like your daughter has what's known as a *fissured* or *lingual tongue*. It's also medically known by the rather unappealing term *scrotal tongue,* though it affects both girls and boys. Lingual tongue is a quite common, inherited condition. But it's not always noticed until a child is older.

STOP SIGN

STOP In addition to toothbrushing, gently cleaning your child's tongue with a toothbrush or tongue scraper or brush can help keep it free from bacterial and yeast infections. It can also help keep a baby's breath smelling fresh.

Although usually benign, the grooves in the tongue can fill up with bacteria, leading to halitosis and other oral problems. Practicing good oral hygiene can help prevent these problems.

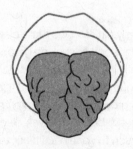

LINGUAL (SCROTAL) TONGUE

HEART-SHAPED TONGUE

Q: *My 6-month-old granddaughter has an indentation on the tip of her tongue, making it look like a heart. Is this normal and will it affect her speech?*

A: Most tongue tips are pointed or oval. A heart-shaped tongue (aka *bifid tongue*), which may also be described as having a W-shaped tip, can be a perfectly normal variation. However, it can also be a telltale sign of a condition commonly called *tongue tie* (aka *ankyloglossia*). Tongue tie is the result of a tight or short *frenulum,* the small piece of skin that attaches the tongue to the floor of the mouth.

> **SIGN OF THE TIMES**
>
> French midwives used to keep one fingernail long so that they could cut the frenulum, the membrane under a baby's tongue. They believed this would make it easier for the baby to nurse.

As the name implies, babies with tongue tie have a limited ability to move their tongues from side to side or up and down, and may even have trouble licking their lips. In fact, a classic sign is their inability to stick out their tongues. They may also have trouble "cupping," that is, wrapping their tongue around a nipple, finger, or other object placed in their mouths. As a result, tongue tie can interfere with sucking milk from a breast or bottle, or eating solid foods.

And because of its restricted movement, a tied tongue can't easily push food around the mouth toward the throat. This increases the risk of cavities, gum disease, and bad breath. Tongue tie can affect a child's speech as well.

The good news is that for many children with this condition the frenulum will eventually stretch or the child will learn to adapt, sometimes with the help of speech therapy. In rare cases when tongue tie seriously interferes with nursing, eating, or speaking, surgery may be recommended.

SMOOTH TONGUE

Q: *Our baby girl's tongue seems unusually smooth—it doesn't have the little bumps that her older sister's tongue has. Can this be a sign of something serious?*

A: A healthy tongue should be rosy and silky soft, with uniform bumps. If a baby has a smooth tongue, it can be a red flag of a vitamin deficiency, especially vitamin B_{12} and folic acid. If a tongue is both smooth and very pale, it can signal an iron deficiency. A smooth tongue may also be a telltale sign of *celiac disease* (aka *sprue* and *malabsorption syndrome*), an intestinal disorder in which the body cannot adequately absorb nutrients. Children with celiac disease can't digest the protein gluten, which is found in wheat, rye, and barley products.

These and other nutritional deficiencies can cause the tongue to lose its coarse covering, become very tender, and even shrink. The good news is that nutritional supplements usually smooth out the problem and restore the tongue to its healthy state.

WARNING SIGN

If your baby's tongue changes color—from its normal pink to strawberry red with white spots or to beefy red—it can be the earliest warning sign of scarlet fever. The good news is that scarlet fever, which was once a major cause of heart valve damage, can today be treated successfully with antibiotics.

TRAVELING TONGUE PATCHES

Q: *I just noticed that my son's tongue is covered with irregular, discolored, rough patches that seem to come and go. Should I be concerned?*

A: Your son may have a fairly common condition called *geographic tongue* (aka *benign migratory glossitis*). The hallmarks of geographic tongue are irregular areas that make the tongue look like a map, hence its name. The patches also seem to travel from place to place: They pop up in one spot and then disappear, only to arrive on another part of the tongue.

Geographic tongue is a harmless condition that tends to run in families. Some children may also have a fissured tongue. (See **A Groovy Tongue,** above.) The patches, which can be white, red, rough, or smooth, are usually painless. But eating hot or spicy food may cause some discomfort.

TREMBLING TONGUE

Q: *I realize that babies' tongues often tremble when they cry, but our daughter's tongue trembles at other times as well. Should we be concerned?*

A: While a tongue tremor in a baby can be perfectly normal, it may also be a sign of a condition called *essential tremor (ET)*. This fairly common movement disorder that usually strikes adults is sometimes seen in children as young as a year old. ET tends to affect more boys than girls and often runs in families. It can cause tremors in the hands, arms, legs, and voice box as well. While the tremors may slowly worsen over time, ET is usually harmless and doesn't require any treatment.

Some babies with ET may have *shuddering spells,* benign attacks in which the child shivers uncontrollably for brief periods (see Chapter 7). In rare cases, a trembling tongue can occur with certain neurological or other disorders. These include *dystonia* (involuntary muscle contractions), *hyperthyroidism* (see Chapter 3), and *Wilson's disease,* a genetic condition in which there is an excess amount of copper in the body. However, with these conditions, more obvious and disturbing signs would also be present.

> **SIGN OF THE TIMES**
>
> According to an American old wives' tale, a baby with a large tongue was bound to be a good singer.

A BABY'S GUMS

A baby's gums are probably of much less interest to parents than any other part of the baby's mouth. But they shouldn't be. They're immensely important during infancy, helping babies latch on to their mothers' nipples and baby bottles. And from toddlerhood onward, the aptly named gums, along with bone, are the glue that holds the teeth in place.

Gums get a lot of wear and tear. In infancy, they do much of the work that the teeth will later do by chewing—or, more accurately, gumming—food. A baby's gums are also exposed to all kinds of assaults from food, fluids, bacteria, and biting. A peek at a baby's gums may provide clues as to what went on in the womb, what's going on now, or what may erupt in the future.

MILKY MOUTH

Q: *My neighbor's baby has thrush. What is it and can my toddler get it if he plays with her?*

A: Thrush, medically known as *candidiasis* or *candida infection,* is a yeast infection of the mouth. The yeast that causes it is everywhere in the environment. In general, thrush is very common in infants. Although rarely seen during the first week of life, it's most common during the next several.

The hallmarks of thrush are irregular white or mother-of-pearl-like patches that *cannot* be wiped away. It usually shows up on the gums, the inside of the lips and cheek, or on the tongue, where it's often mistaken for milk residue.

Some children, especially babies who have a diaper rash caused by yeast, are at greater risk for thrush than others. Thrush can be a reaction to certain prescribed drugs such as steroids or antibiotics. Because antibiotics can pass through breast milk, a nursing baby can get thrush if his or her mother is taking antibiotics. And mothers who have a vaginal yeast infection when pregnant can pass it along to their babies during delivery.

The reverse is also true. If a nursing baby has thrush, he or she can pass it on to his or her mother's nipples when breast-feeding. Unless both mother and baby are treated, the infection can ping-pong between them. Babies with thrush may also spread it to other children through shared bottles, pacifiers, teething rings, and toys that they put in their mouths. Fortunately, thrush can be easily treated with a simple antifungal medication.

CROOKED GUMS

Q: *My new granddaughter's gums look uneven. I'm concerned her teeth may grow in crooked, but my daughter says it's nothing to worry about. Is she right?*

A: An uneven gum line is usually the result of an abnormally shaped jaw—medically called *positional deformity of the jaw*. This rare occurrence results from constant pressure on a baby's chin in the womb. For example, the baby's developing chin may have rested for a long time against his or her own shoulder or against the mother's pelvis. This is similar to the head molding that's seen in newborns (see Chapter 1). The baby's cheek on the unaffected side might be fuller than the other. The good news is that positional deformity of the jaw is usually both benign and temporary. It almost always straightens out on its own, and the teeth will come in normally.

TINY GUM DOTS

Q: *For the past few months, our baby has had several very tiny whitish-yellowish dots on her gums. I thought they were budding teeth, but they haven't grown. What could they be?*

A: The dots you describe sound like they are a very common, benign condition medically known as *Bohn's nodules*. In fact, about 80% of newborns have these gingival (gum) cysts, as they're sometimes called. When they're found on the roof of a baby's mouth, they're called *Epstein's pearls*.

It's not unusual for these small lumps to be mistaken for budding teeth. But they're actually small fluid-filled growths that are the oral equivalent to *milia,* more commonly known as baby acne (see Chapter 8). Both the pimples and pearls are likely to disappear on their own as the baby gets older.

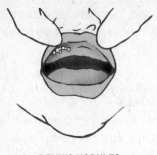

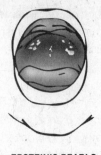

BOHN'S NODULES   **EPSTEIN'S PEARLS**

BAD BABY BREATH

Q: My 18-month-old son has a playmate with bad breath. Could he possibly have gum disease?

A: Just like adults, babies and toddlers can have bad breath, sometimes from the same causes. A dry mouth is often to blame. Once saliva dries up, the naturally occurring bacteria in the mouth tend to overgrow. The result: bad breath, also known as *halitosis* or, more currently, *oral malodor.*

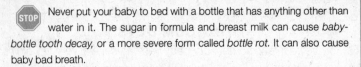

STOP SIGN

STOP Never put your baby to bed with a bottle that has anything other than water in it. The sugar in formula and breast milk can cause *baby-bottle tooth decay,* or a more severe form called *bottle rot.* It can also cause baby bad breath.

There are a host of reasons why a baby's mouth can become dry, and mouth breathing is a prime culprit. Babies who suck their thumbs, pacifiers, security blankets, or toys may also wind up with a mouth that's dry because their saliva ends up on these objects rather than staying in their mouths. Plus the saliva left on these sucked-on items may dry up and harbor germs. When the child puts them back into his or her mouth, these germs can cause bad breath.

Bad breath can also be a telling sign that a baby has oral thrush (see **Milky Mouth,** above) or another infection in the mouth, teeth, throat, tonsils, sinuses, or even ears. These infections can cause babies to breathe through their mouths. (Babies usually breathe only through their noses during the first 4 to 6 months of life.) Bad baby breath can also signal allergies and postnasal drip. And it can be an important warning sign that a baby has a foreign object lodged in his or her nose, a fairly common occurrence in this age group. (See Chapter 5.)

Chronic bad breath is a hallmark of *tonsil stones,* medically known as *tonsilloliths* or *calculi*. If a tonsil has lots of deep nooks and crannies, food, bacteria, mucus, and dead cells can get trapped, forming these unsavory stones.

Finally, a baby can have foul breath from frequently spitting up, which may be caused by acid reflux (aka heartburn or gastrointestinal reflux).

A BABY'S TEETH

In a manner of speaking, teething actually begins in the womb as early as 6 weeks' gestation when the first teeth begin to form. But it's not until a baby is about 6 months old that these teeth begin to emerge. For a nursing mother, a little nip on her nipple may be the first sign that her baby's baby teeth are making an appearance.

Many parents anticipate the arrival of their baby's first teeth with mixed emotions. Teething is an exciting milestone on a baby's road to toddlerhood and beyond. On the other hand, most parents dread the crankiness, drooling, and long nights they may have to spend soothing their teething babies. Throughout the ages, parents and physicians have determinedly debated whether a fever or other troubles ranging from diarrhea to convulsions heralded the onset of tooth eruptions. In some medical and social circles, the controversy continues to this day.

Babies have 20 *primary teeth,* commonly referred to as milk teeth. Rather than being milky white, they're normally off-white or ivory. These first teeth are ultimately replaced by 32

SIGN OF THE TIMES

Exchanging lost baby teeth for gifts is an old European tradition dating back to Viking days. These tiny teeth were believed to ward off witches and evil spirits. The legend of the Tooth Fairy lives to this day. A child will tuck a lost tooth under a pillow anxiously awaiting a coin or small gift left by the Tooth Fairy. In the United States these days, the Tooth Fairy is paying about $2 per tooth, according to a national financial magazine.

SIGNS OF THE TIMES

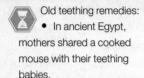

Old teething remedies:
- In ancient Egypt, mothers shared a cooked mouse with their teething babies.
- In ancient Rome, the first tooth of a horse to fall out, a wolf's tooth, or a viper's brain or teeth were made into amulets and strung around babies' necks.
- In 17th-century England, coral was made into a baby necklace or hung on a baby's crib.
- In medieval France, babies were given a sachet housing a paw of a mole that had been tortured and decapitated. The mole's pain was supposed to supplant the baby's.
- Leeches latched on as a cure in 19th-century Europe and the United States. They were placed on a baby's gums, which were also sometimes lanced.
- The longest lasting hare-brained remedy was literally a hare's brain. As early as the 1st century and continuing through the 17th century, hares' brains were fed to teething babies or applied to their gums in various Western nations.

permanent teeth, a process that can take more than 20 years.

Teeth perform many functions, from chewing food to helping to form words. And how they grow can affect everything from the shape of a baby's face to his or her smile.

TINY TEETH

Q: *We just came back from visiting my sister's infant son and noticed that he already has teeth. Is this normal?*

A: Normally teeth start coming in when a baby is about 6 months old. When present at birth, they're medically referred to as *natal teeth*. In these cases, usually only 2 or 3 small, brownish teeth are seen on the bottom gums. Natal teeth are quite rare and are more common in babies born with a cleft lip or palate. Sometimes they occur in babies who have more severe congenital disorders, but in these cases there would be other more obvious signs.

Because natal teeth are not very secure in a baby's gums, they're usually removed to prevent them from being dislodged and swallowed.

If a baby's teeth appear during the first few weeks of life rather than at birth, he or she may have an even rarer condition called *neonatal teeth*. This type of early tooth development tends to run in families. Although usually harmless, sharp neonatal teeth sometimes irritate a baby's tender tongue and cause an ulcer, medically called *Riga-Fede disease*. This is an unfortunate moniker because it's not a disease at all. The ulcer can, however, interfere with breast- or bottle-feeding. Depending on how troublesome it is, treatment ranges from the conservative to surgical removal of the offending tooth or teeth.

The early appearance of teeth is usually not a sign of a medical problem. That said, children who have neonatal teeth are more likely to go through early puberty than others. Neonatal teeth have also been associated with *hyperthyroidism,* the overproduction of thyroid hormone (see Chapter 3), and certain genetic conditions such as *Sotos syndrome,* in which children tend to grow quickly (their adult height is, however, usually normal) and have other facial anomalies.

For the most part, both natal and neonatal teeth are normal primary teeth—once they're lost, they're replaced by permanent teeth. If the early teeth appear in the back of the mouth, dental treatment may be needed to ensure that there's enough space for the rest of the child's permanent teeth to come in.

TARDY TEETH

Q: *Our baby girl is 18 months old and she hasn't gotten any teeth yet. All our other children started teething be-*

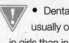

SIGNIFICANT FACTS

- Dental development usually occurs a bit earlier in girls than in boys.
- Boys have slightly larger teeth and roots than girls.
- Overweight babies tend to get their teeth earlier than normal-weight ones.

SIGNS OF THE TIMES

- A baby boy in ancient Rome was given the name Manius Curius Dentatus because he was born with teeth.
- In medieval Europe it was believed that babies born with teeth were destined to achieve great eminence.
- In 15th-century England, King Richard III was born with teeth and, according to Shakespeare, "could gnaw a crust at two hours old."
- In France, some notable noblemen with natal teeth included Cardinal Richelieu, Louis XIV, and Napoleon.

SIGN OF THE TIMES

One in 3 children will get at least 1 cavity in their baby teeth.

SIGN OF THE TIMES

The ancient Mayans believed that if a pregnant woman pocketed a comb in the folds of her skirt, her child would have crooked teeth.

fore their 1st birthdays. Could there be a problem?

A: While there's a wide variation in when babies get their teeth, most babies start getting teeth at about 6 months of age. Your daughter may be experiencing *delayed teething*—medically defined as teeth erupting 6 or more months later than usual. It sometimes runs in families.

Delayed teething—or even teeth that come in asymmetrically—can be a warning sign of thyroid, pituitary, or other hormonal disorders. Children who were born prematurely or have certain obvious genetic disorders, such as Down syndrome or dwarfism, may also experience delayed teething.

By the age of 3, most children have all of their primary teeth. Having few or no teeth at all at this age is very rare and can be a warning sign of *ectodermal dysplasia* (*ED*), a group of rare genetic conditions in which the skin, hair, nails, teeth, and/or sweat glands don't develop normally. ED can also result in misshapen teeth, particularly pegged or pointed ones. In some cases, this condition is apparent at birth because of some more obvious problems, such as a cleft palate and lip. In other cases, it's detected only when a baby's teeth don't develop normally. While ED is not curable, there are many treatments available to address some of its complications.

DISCOLORED TEETH

Q: My 8-month-old nephew's new teeth look stained. My sister's pretty fussy about dental hygiene. Why would his teeth be discolored?

A: It's not that unusual for babies or toddlers to have discolored teeth, which can be the result of any number of factors. For example, a gray or brownish stain may be a sign that the baby's mother had an illness and/or took the antibiotic tetracycline during pregnancy. The staining

causes teeth to look mottled, which is due to actual deposits of antibiotic in the teeth. Because tetracycline and tetracycline-like antibiotics
can cause permanent teeth to come in stained, they're not usually given
to children younger than 12 years of age. Babies who've had a high
fever during the time their teeth were developing may wind up with discolored permanent teeth.

Distinctive dark dots or spots on a
baby's teeth can be a telltale sign of
a condition aptly called *black stain,*
which is caused by excessive bacteria in the saliva, a hereditary trait. And
gray-black teeth can be due to iron
supplements.

Discolored teeth in children can also

be a warning sign of damage to the tooth enamel called *dental fluorosis*. This is caused by excess fluoride from water, rinses, toothpaste, or
supplements. Tooth color changes can range from white spots to brown
and black stains; the discoloration also gives the teeth a mottled look.
Severe dental fluorosis can permanently damage tooth enamel and lead
to cavities.

If a baby's tooth or teeth look iridescent or have a black-and-blue
appearance, it can be a telltale sign of a physical injury. The darkening
results from damage to the tooth's pulp or nerve. Trauma to a baby
tooth can actually cause discoloration to the permanent tooth when it
comes in.

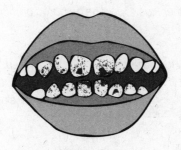

DENTAL FLUOROSIS

BLUE-TINGED TEETH

Q: My toddler's teeth have a bluish tint, and a few have even broken off. My grandmother had weak teeth too. Could my daughter have inherited this tendency?

SPEAKING OF SIGNS

White sugar, black teeth.
—Croatian proverb

A: It is possible that your daughter has a very rare genetic tooth disorder called *dentinogenesis imperfecta* (*DI*). The typical signs of DI are bluish gray, brown, or other odd-colored teeth that fracture easily. Although DI makes both the primary and permanent teeth susceptible to decay, the good news is that it doesn't affect any other part of the body.

MOUTH-RELATED BEHAVIOR

YAWNING A LOT

Q: I babysit for a toddler who yawns a lot, even when he's well rested and playing with other kids. Could he be bored or might there be something wrong with him?

A: It's not unusual for babies to yawn a lot. Indeed, they do so in the womb as early as 12 weeks after conception. Most babies tend to yawn before going to sleep at night or for naps, and some yawn when they wake up.

SIGNIFICANT FACT

 Mammals, birds, reptiles, and even fish yawn.

Babies sometimes do get bored, especially if they're not getting enough stimulation from play or interaction with others. This may lead to sleepiness and yawning. Yawning is also notoriously contagious. So if you or the other people around the baby yawn a lot, he may just be following suit.

There is some debate, though, as to whether children under 2 years old can "catch a yawn." Contagious yawning is believed to be a sign of empathy, and most young babies are not yet capable of empathy. Interestingly, both contagious yawning and empathy are rare—or at least very delayed—in autistic children.

For the most part, yawning is a benign albeit boring activity. In rare cases, however, excessive yawning can signal some medical conditions ranging from infections to such neurological problems as multiple sclerosis.

SIGNIFICANT FACT

Contagious yawning is not only a human trait; it's also been spotted in chimpanzees. And it's not only primates that mimic one another's yawns. Recently researchers found that some dogs will copycat a human's yawn with a yawn of their own.

SIGN OF THE TIMES

Ancient Roman doctors believed that yawning in babies was responsible for the high infant mortality rate. As a preventive measure, doctors instructed mothers to cover the mouths of their yawning babies.

DROOLING A LOT

Q: *My 3-month-old drools like a spout. I don't think she's teething because she's too young and not very cranky. What else could be causing this?*

A: It's very natural for babies to start drooling at your daughter's age. Before 2 to 3 months of age, babies don't produce saliva—ergo, no slobbering. Some think that saliva starts to spew just in time to help babies digest solid foods. And until a baby's ability to swallow is perfected, the saliva will continue to flow. Indeed, some babies drool so much that their lips and chins develop a rash from it.

SPEAKING OF SIGNS

If you were to open up a baby's head—and I am not for a moment suggesting that you should—you would find nothing but an enormous drool gland.

—Dave Barry, humor writer

SPEAKING OF SIGNS

> To cure slobbering in a baby, take it to a creek, catch three minnows, hold the first minnow by the tail while drawing it through the baby's mouth, and then let the fish flop back into the creek.

— Illinois folklore

Both drooling and irritability are, indeed, common signs of teething. But most people don't realize that babies as young as 3 months old do sometimes teethe (see **Tiny Teeth,** above), and they're not always irritable. The drooling can run for some time before a tooth actually breaks through the gums. Other signs of teething are bumpy gums and tiny openings in the gums where teeth will soon emerge.

On the other hand, drooling sometimes signals acid (gastrointestinal) reflux, which is the backup of food or stomach acids into the esophagus. Because the stomach acids actually burn and irritate the back of the throat, the baby may have trouble swallowing and may drool more. In addition to saliva, the drool may contain these regurgitated stomach contents.

WARNING SIGN

While most babies occasionally have bouts of hiccups, a baby who hiccups excessively may have *gastroesophageal reflux disease (GERD)*, a severe form of acid reflux (heartburn). In children, GERD is often associated with a variety of other medical conditions, including respiratory and nutritional problems.

STUFFING STUFF IN THE MOUTH

Q: *My 20-month-old puts everything in her mouth, from her thumb to her toys and the tip of her blankie. Can this be a sign of insecurity or some other problem?*

A: Putting things in the mouth is a very natural part of being a toddler. Aptly called *mouthing,* it is a way in which babies explore their world. They sometimes pretend to eat by substituting toys for food. Chewing on various objects also helps soothe the gums of a teething toddler. Of course, the danger here is that babies may accidentally swallow and/or choke on the different doodads that they deposit in their mouths.

Some children who frequently shove strange things in their mouths may have a medical condition called *pica*. Children with this disorder frequently ingest nonfood items such as dirt, paint chips, or hair (see Chapter 2). Pica is somewhat more common in children with *sickle-cell anemia* than in other children. Interestingly, this condition is actually fairly common in pregnant women. Pica in both children and adults is thought to be associated with an iron or zinc deficiency.

> **SIGNIFICANT FACT**
>
> The word *pica* is the Latin word for "magpie." Magpies are birds famous for eating virtually anything they can get their little beaks on.

NOCTURNAL NOISES

Q: *I can hear my toddler grinding his teeth at night. I know that adults often do this when they're tense. Why would a child do this?*

A: Some children do indeed grind their teeth, medically called *bruxism*. One in every 3 children will grind their teeth at some point during childhood. In some children, it can be a warning sign of a misalignment of the top and bottom teeth, which can cause children to move their teeth back and forth. Teeth grinding may also signal an imbalance in ear pressure, in which case the jaw movement may help relieve the discomfort. And as with adults, bruxism in children can be a sign of tension, anger, or fear.

> **SPEAKING OF SIGNS**
>
> *Adam and Eve had many advantages, but the principal one was that they escaped teething.*
>
> —Mark Twain, *Pudd'nhead Wilson,* 1894

Most children, like adults, grind their teeth when they are sleeping at night, a time when it can be very grating on their parents' ears. In fact, the grinding can be so intense that parents have said they can hear the noise from another room. Bruxism is more common in children who have other nighttime and sleep problems, called *parasomnias,* such as bed-wetting, muscle cramps, and sleep talking. Regardless of the cause, teeth guards are sometimes recommended to help cut down on the grinding. Guards are particularly good at preventing permanent damage to permanent teeth.

A BABY'S VOICE

Gurgling, cooing, babbling, and uttering noises other than crying are all key vocal activities in babies. Indeed, babbling is a critical step in speech development. A baby's voice rhythms and other speech patterns can say a great deal about a child's language development. A voice that sounds harsh or hoarse, or too loud, soft, or nasal, may signal anything from a cold to a hearing problem or a voice disorder. And a very unusual voice can sound the alarm for a developmental and/or neurological disorder.

A RASPY VOICE

Q: Our toddler's voice always sounds hoarse. He doesn't have a cold, so what else could be causing this?

A: There are many reasons why a child may have a hoarse or raspy voice, medically known as *dysphonia*. Even if your son doesn't currently have a cold, he could have lingering *laryngitis* from a previous one. Temporary hoarseness can also occur when babies strain their voices after crying or laughing loudly.

Vocal cord nodules, noncancerous growths on the vocal cords, are the most common cause of hoarseness in children. These benign growths are usually due to voice abuse from screaming, shouting, or screeching for prolonged periods. Not surprisingly, boys are at increased risk, as are children who live in large families. With voice rest and sometimes voice therapy, the hoarseness usually clears up.

Dysphonia can also be a sign of a variety of chronic medical problems, including allergies, postnasal drip, asthma, GERD, or thyroid disorders. Treatment of the underlying problem, and sometimes voice therapy, usually restores the voice to normal.

In very rare cases, dysphonia can signal other types of benign, or even malignant, tumors in the throat, larynx, or elsewhere in the upper respiratory tract. In these cases, surgery is usually necessary.

> **SIGN OF THE TIMES**
>
> In medieval Europe babies were expected to talk when they had all their teeth, usually around the age of 2. One cure for slow-to-speak babies was a concoction of salt, honey, frankincense, and licorice rubbed on the baby's tongue.

STAMMERING WHEN SPEAKING

Q: *Our adopted 2-year-old son has started to stutter. I thought only older children stutter. Can he outgrow this or will he always have a problem?*

A: It's not unusual for children between the ages of 2 and 5 to stutter. The stuttering, medically known as *speech disfluency* or *dysfluency,* often begins when they start speaking fluently, and their brains are working faster and more efficiently than their tongues. If your son was born into a non-English-speaking family, his disfluency may be caused by his efforts to adjust to his new language.

Boys are 3 times more likely than girls to be stutterers, but the good news is that most will outgrow this *pseudostuttering,* as it's sometimes called, in 3 to 4 years. Children who start stuttering after the age of 8 are more likely to continue into adulthood. Speech disfluencies are very rare in adults, though, affecting less than 1%.

Although the cause of stuttering is unknown and it's unclear whether or not genes are involved, it often runs in families. In some cases, there may be a neurological component, but stuttering is rarely a sign of a medical or psychological problem. However, emotional factors do play a role: Stut-

> **SIGNIFICANT FACT**
>
> Recent research has found that young children with speech problems often have feeding difficulties. Other signs that were frequently found in children with speech problems were drooling, acid reflux, and bruxism.

tering often becomes worse when a child is overly excited, stressed, or tired. Interestingly, most stutterers are able to talk to themselves or sing without stammering.

There's debate as to whether stuttering in young children should be ignored or treated with speech therapy. Most experts do recommend that if the problem persists for more than 5 or 6 months, or if it's causing the child to become overly self-conscious, a speech evaluation is in order.

SIGNING OFF

An important part of a newborn's examination is an exploration of the mouth. In addition to making sure that the baby's mouth is clear of mucus and secretions that can hamper breathing or cause choking, the doctor will check the infant's mouth, both inside and out, for abnormalities. Each time a baby goes for a checkup, his or her mouth will again be thoroughly evaluated.

STOP SIGN

 The first dental visit should take place at or near a child's 1st birthday, according to the major medical pediatric and dental associations.

However, certain mouth-related problems may occur in between well-baby visits that call for an immediate call to the doctor or a trip to the doctor's office. For example, if your baby has had an injury to the mouth—especially if it results in broken teeth—call your baby's pediatrician or dentist or take your baby in for a visit. And some mouth-related problems may even require a trip to the emergency room.

GO TO THE EMERGENCY ROOM OR CALL 911 IF YOUR BABY:

- Has profuse and prolonged bleeding from the mouth, lips, or gums
- Vomits blood
- Suddenly develops a swollen tongue and/or lips and is having trouble breathing or swallowing
- Suddenly develops blue lips and other parts of his or her

body (cyanosis) *and* is having trouble breathing or appears very sick

- Has swallowed household cleaning fluids or other products
- Has swallowed a nonfood item, especially a button battery, which can cause permanent damage within an hour

If your baby has something stuck in the throat, immediately call 911. Your baby's pediatrician or other healthcare provider can usually treat most mouth-related problems. But in some cases, a child may be referred to such specialists as an ear, nose, and throat (ENT) doctor (*otorhinolaryngologist*), allergist, pediatric dentist, and/or speech therapist.

Chapter 7

YOUR BABY'S TORSO AND LIMBS

Children, you are very little,
And your bones are very brittle;
If you would grow great and stately,
You must try to walk sedately.
—Robert Louis Stevenson,
A Child's Garden of Verses, 1885

AT BIRTH, A BABY'S HEAD usually arrives first, giving the parents an exciting glimpse of what their newborn looks like. But it's not until the baby's torso completely emerges that parents discover the size, shape, and sex of their baby (that is, unless the mother had amniocentesis or another prenatal diagnostic test).

While a baby's head houses the brain and 4 of the 5 senses, the baby's torso is host to the heart, lungs, stomach, and all the other vital organs. It is also where some of the more interesting external parts are found—from the breasts and belly button to the buttocks and genitals (which are covered in Chapter 9).

So while new parents may be more excited by their baby's smiling face than they are by his or her arms, hands, fingers, legs, feet, and toes, these body parts loom large in the life of every growing child. Babies' arms hug their moms and dads, and their tiny hands grasp their bottles, toys, and, most endearingly, their parents' fingers. They use their own little fingers as pacifiers and as tools for exploring new objects and food.

Navels have been the subject of fascinated contemplation by babies and parents alike. And last but not least, legs and feet let the baby lunge forth into the world as an upright, if sometimes tottering, toddler.

Besides being essential to physical functioning, a baby's torso and extremities also provide parents with a whole host of helpful hints about the state of their baby's health.

BABY BOSOMS

BUDDING BREASTS IN BABY GIRLS

Q: *My 1-month-old daughter has quite large breasts for a baby. What could be causing it?*

A: Enlarged breasts at or soon after birth are an extremely common, benign occurrence. In fact, about 90% of newborn girls *and* boys have tiny breasts. (See **Budding Breasts in Baby Boys,** below.)

Enlarged breasts in newborns are caused by the large amounts of estrogen that pass from mother to baby in the womb. In some cases, the estrogen can continue to circulate in the baby's body for several months following birth. When this happens, the body reacts as though it's entering puberty: The breasts temporarily enlarge and may even leak (see **Leaky Nipples,** below). No treatment is needed; the breasts will usually revert to normal within 2 to 3 weeks after birth, or longer in breast-fed babies. In baby girls, they may stay enlarged for up to 24 months, a condition referred to as *premature thelarche.* Although usually benign, premature thelarche can be a warning sign of *hypothyroidism* (underactive thyroid) or even ovarian cysts.

SIGN OF THE TIMES

Many rituals revolving around cutting the umbilical cord persisted into the 20th century. In parts of Europe and the United States, it was believed that in baby boys, the length of the remaining cord would determine the ultimate length of the boy's penis. Another common belief was that if the cord was cut too short, the baby would be a bed-wetter.

SIGNS OF THE TIMES

- The Greek word for "navel," *omphalos,* refers to the center of the world.
- Hawaiians use the same word—*piko*—for the navel and the umbilical cord, which they used to believe connected babies to their ancestors.
- In Italy, legend has it that the navel of Venus, the goddess of love, is the model for the popular pasta tortellini.

Any baby girl with enlarged breasts should also be monitored for acne, pubic and/or underarm hair, vaginal bleeding, and rapid growth— the hallmarks of *precocious puberty*. (Boys can also have precocious puberty; they may have an enlarged penis or testicles in addition to the other signs of early puberty. See Chapter 9.) Precocious puberty is usually caused by a hormonal disorder. Treatment typically involves hormones or other medications.

WARNING SIGN

A recent study in the *New England Journal of Medicine* found that using products that contain lavender or tea tree oil can cause enlarged breasts (*gynecomastia*) in young boys. These are often in soaps, shampoos, and lotions. The good news is that once these essential oils are no longer used, the breasts return to normal.

Both premature thelarche and precocious puberty are more common among children of African and Hispanic descent than among whites. The highest incidence has been found in girls born and raised in Puerto Rico; researchers believe that environmental toxins are responsible. These conditions have also been linked to exposure to estrogen-containing skin and hair products, poultry, soy-based infant formula, and even fennel-containing preparations, which are often used to help eliminate gas and regulate bowel function. Although baby boys who are exposed to estrogen-containing products may have enlarged breasts, their genitals will not be impacted.

WARNING SIGN

Any baby boy or girl whose breasts remain enlarged for several months should be evaluated by a pediatrician or pediatric endocrinologist as soon as possible.

BUDDING BREASTS IN BABY BOYS

Q: *I'm worried about my 3-month-old grandson. His breasts are quite large. Neither of my two sons had breasts as babies. Could something be wrong?*

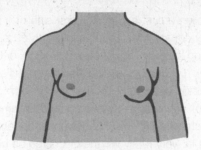

GYNECOMASTIA IN BABY BOY

A: Breasts in infant boys, called *neonatal gynecomastia,* is an extremely common condition. Like breasts in baby girls (see **Budding Breasts in Baby Girls,** above), breasts in baby boys is usually a normal, benign condition that's the result of large amounts of estrogen passing from mother to baby in the womb.

Neonatal gynecomastia usually disappears within 1 to 3 weeks after birth, but it can sometimes persist for several months. Occasionally the enlarged breasts may leak milk. (See **Leaky Nipples,** below.) If a boy's breasts remain swollen after his first birthday, he should be given a complete medical evaluation by a pediatric endocrinologist.

> **WARNING SIGN**
>
> If your newborn has swollen breasts, don't try to express milk from them through massage or any other means. This may prolong or worsen the condition and can also cause an infection, such as neonatal mastitis, or even a cystic tumor in the mammary gland.

Although enlarged breasts may be nothing more than a telltale sign that a baby boy is obese, it could also signal any number of hormonal conditions, such as *hypogonadism* (aka *Klinefelter syndrome*) (see Chapter 9). Treatment of these conditions often involves hormonal therapy. In very rare cases, breasts in boys can be a warning sign of an adrenal tumor, which usually requires surgical removal.

ONE SWOLLEN BREAST

Q: *Our newborn daughter's left breast is swollen, but her right one is normal. What could have caused this?*

A: A single swollen breast can be the first sign of a breast infection, medically called *neonatal mastitis*. This infection usually occurs in full-term infants during the first 2 to 3 weeks after birth, but rarely later than 2 months of age. In young babies, it affects both girls and boys equally, but when it occurs in older babies, it's more common in girls.

Other signs of neonatal mastitis are a red, inflamed breast that's warm to the touch, swollen lymph nodes under the arm, and pus oozing from the nipple. Very rarely will the discharge be bloody. Many babies who develop this type of breast infection, which is usually caused by the *staph* bacterium, will also have a diaper rash or other skin infection caused by the same bug. Neonatal mastitis is usually treated with antibiotics.

In some cases, the infection will cause an abscess to form, which may need to be aspirated or drained and treated with antibiotics. Unfortunately, in the most severe cases, the infection and the subsequent lancing of the abscess may cause permanent loss of some breast tissue, which can become a cosmetic concern later in life.

WARNING SIGN

There have been recent reports of neonatal mastitis leading to serious breast abscesses caused by methicillin-resistant *Staphylococcus aureus* (*MRSA*). As its name implies, this type of staph infection is becoming increasingly difficult to cure with antibiotics. Unfortunately, MRSA infections can sometimes be fatal.

Alternatively, a single swollen breast may signal *mammary duct ectasia,* a usually benign blockage of the milk ducts. In babies this is a very rare condition that can affect both boys and girls. The fluid in the blocked ducts can back up, and if it's darkly colored, the area under the baby's nipple may develop a blue tinge. (This condition is commonly called *blue breast*.) Mammary duct ectasia can also cause nipple discharge, which may be sticky or even bloody. The color of the discharge may vary depending on the different substances in the milk ducts. Mammary duct ectasia can also increase a baby's risk of a breast infection. The good news is that the blockage and discharge usually resolve on their own in 6 to 9 months.

TRIPLE BREASTS

Q: *I've noticed a breastlike bump on our baby daughter's chest just below one of her nipples. What can it be?*

A: Your daughter—along with up to 5% of newborn baby girls *and* boys—may have extra breast tissue, a condition referred to as *polymastia*. Although fairly rare, extra breasts, called *supernumerary breasts,* sometimes run in families. The extra breast may even have a nipple and/or an areola. (See **Triple Nipples,** below.) Most of these mammary marvels are so small they're not noticed until they start to develop during puberty.

Supernumerary breasts usually form along the *milk line,* an imaginary line extending from under the nipples to the groin. But they have also been spotted on other parts of the body, including the buttocks, neck, shoulders, and back.

For the most part, supernumerary breasts, and nipples for that matter, are only a cosmetic problem. In rare cases, polymastia has been linked to defects in the kidneys and other organs. And any problem that can occur in a normal breast, including cancer, can occur in the extra one as well. If the extra breast causes your child discomfort, secretes milk, or even causes undue embarrassment, surgery is an option.

NEWBORN NIPPLES

LEAKY NIPPLES

Q: *When I was visiting my newborn nephew, I noticed some discharge from his nipples on his T-shirt. My sister said it was nothing to worry about, but I'm concerned. Should I be?*

A: It's not unusual for a newborn boy or girl to have nipple discharge from one or both breasts. In fact, about 5% of newborn babies have leaky nipples. The fluid can be clear, but it's more frequently milky, which may be one reason it's colorfully referred to as *witch's milk*.

This harmless discharge is caused when the mother's hormones, which are quite high in the last trimester of pregnancy, cross the placenta and stimulate the baby's breast tissue. The leaking usually lasts for only a few weeks, but sometimes it can continue for longer. (See **Budding Breasts in Baby Boys,** above.)

If the discharge is bloody or varies in color, it may be a sign of mammary duct ectasia, a benign blockage of the milk duct. (See **One Swollen Breast,** above.) While it's distressing to parents, bloody nipple discharge in infants is rare and nearly always benign. It generally resolves on its own within a few months.

Sometimes the mother's hormones will cause not only nipple discharge but the baby's breasts to enlarge as well. (See **Budding Breasts in Baby Girls,** above.) These enlarged breasts may take a few months or even longer to shrink to normal.

TRIPLE NIPPLES

Q: I was babysitting for my 3-month-old niece and I noticed that she has a tiny spot on her side that looks just like a nipple. Is that possible?

A: Having 3 or more nipples, medically known as *polythelia*, isn't that unusual. Indeed, an estimated 5% of boys and girls are born with these *supernumerary nipples* (SNs), as they're called.

Like supernumerary breasts (see **Triple Breasts,** above), these extra nipples are usually found along what's called the "milk line"—the chest or lower abdominal area where the nipples of other mammals are found. But they sometimes appear in more unusual spots, such as on the neck, armpit, or even forehead. These superfluous nipples can look remarkably like normal nipples and in rare cases may actually develop into milk-producing breasts.

While this condition is usually benign, children with multiple nipples may have skeletal deformities and may be at increased risk for certain

---

WARNING SIGN

While an extra nipple or breast is usually nothing to worry about, the presence of only one nipple or breast—an extremely rare anomaly—sometimes occurs with other congenital abnormalities.

medical conditions, including ulcers, migraines, and gallbladder problems. And like extra breasts (see **Triple Breasts,** above), extra nipples can also be a sign of rare genetic kidney and urinary tract defects.

INVISIBLE NIPPLES

Q: My baby granddaughter's nipples are pushed in. What causes this and could it interfere with her being able to breast-feed her own child when she grows up?

A: It's not uncommon for both girls and boys to be born with one or both nipples turning inward. These *inverted nipples,* as they're called, occur when the tissue that normally pushes the nipple and surrounding area outward fails to do so. In most cases, this tissue will eventually stretch and allow the nipples to extend forward into their normal position. Permanently inverted nipples are rare, but even if your granddaughter's nipples stay inverted, it doesn't mean that she won't be able to breast-feed. There are many effective nursing aids available for women with inverted nipples and other breast-feeding problems.

SUNKEN CHEST

Q: My 3-month-old godson's chest looks somewhat caved in. What could this mean?

A: If your godson's chest always has a sunken appearance (when he both inhales *and* exhales), he might have what's medically known as *pectus excavatum*. Commonly referred to as a *funnel chest*, and sometimes as *cobbler's chest*, this is a fairly rare anatomical abnormality in which the breastbone curves inward rather than outward. It's caused by an overgrowth of the connective tissue that joins the ribs to the breastbone, and is usually noticed at birth or shortly thereafter. Funnel chest often runs in families, and while it's sometimes seen in girls, it's 3 to 4 times more common in boys.

In some cases, funnel chest is benign and unrelated to any other physical problems and is no more than a cosmetic concern. Some children with this condition, however, have certain other bone disorders, including

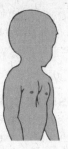

PECTUS EXCAVATUM (FUNNEL CHEST)

scoliosis (curvature of the spine) and *dwarfism,* a genetic condition result-ing in short stature. And they may also be at increased risk for a mild heart condition called *mitral valve prolapse.* In rare cases, babies with funnel chest may have *Marfan syndrome* or *Ehlers-Danlos syndrome* (see **Lim-ber Limbs,** below), both of which are genetic connective-tissue disor-ders that can adversely affect many other parts of the body. (Connective tissues are proteins that support the skin, bones, blood vessels, and other organs.)

In severe cases, a concave chest can push against the heart and lungs, restricting blood flow to and from the heart and forcing the lungs to work harder. This can cause breathing difficulties, fatigue, and seri-ous heart problems. In these situations, surgery may be necessary when the child is older.

WARNING SIGN

If a child's chest curves inward only when he or she inhales, it may be a sign of a respiratory problem, such as a nasal obstruction, asthma, or a lung infection. The child should be evaluated by a doctor as soon as pos-sible.

POINTY CHEST

Q: *I'm a nanny for a 2-year-old whose chest juts out. His mother says he has something called "pigeon chest." What is it and is it serious?*

A: *Pigeon* (aka bowed) *chest* is a very rare chest abnormality that mostly affects boys. Medically known as *pectus carinatum,* it's a defor-

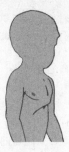

PECTUS CARINATUM (PIGEON CHEST)

mity in which the chest bone and ribs are pushed outward. This makes the chest look rather pointy and protrude like a bird's breast, hence the name "pigeon chest." The cause is unknown, but like funnel chest (see **Sunken Chest,** above), it often runs in families. While it sometimes appears in infancy, pigeon chest doesn't usually show up until early childhood.

Children with pigeon chest are at increased risk for asthma and other respiratory problems. They may have some of the same conditions as children with funnel chest, including scoliosis and mitral valve prolapse, as

> ### SIGNIFICANT FACT
>
> ⚠ Most babies are born with 12 pairs of ribs. But 1 in 20 has an extra set. This harmless occurrence can be seen only on X-ray.

well as other congenital heart problems. Occasionally they will also have vision problems, arthritis, and healing disorders. Treatments for pigeon chest, which often worsens with age, include chest braces and, in severe cases, surgery.

BABY BELLY BUTTON BUMPS, LUMPS, AND STUMPS

BELLY BUTTON BULGE

Q: *I heard that infants can get hernias in their belly buttons. Is that true?*

A: Babies can indeed have *umbilical hernias,* as they're called—in fact, about 1 in 6 babies do!

The abdominal wall normally closes before birth, but when it doesn't close completely, a small bit of tissue can push through and pop out, creating a small pea-sized lump in the belly button—an umbilical hernia. Although this type of abdominal wall defect occurs before a baby is born, parents usually don't begin to notice the hernia until their baby is a few weeks old.

Umbilical hernias are often more apparent when a baby cries, sits up, or strains during a bowel movement. Parents sometimes first notice the hernia when their baby plays with the extra skin around his or her navel. These hernias are different from *inguinal hernias,* a condition in which part of the intestine pushes through the abdominal wall, causing a bulge in a baby's groin, scrotum, or vagina. (See Chapter 9.)

Umbilical hernias are most common in black children, occurring in 1 out of 4. Premature and low-birth-weight babies and babies with underactive thyroids (*hypothyroidism*) are at increased risk, as are babies with certain genetic conditions, including *Down syndrome* and *cystic fibrosis,* an inherited chronic disease that affects the lungs and digestive system.

Most umbilical hernias, especially small ones, will close on their own. Surgical repair may be needed, however, if a hernia is large or if it doesn't close up by the time a child is 3 or 4 years old.

BELLY BUTTON STUMP

Q: After my new grandson's umbilical cord fell off, he still had a piece of pink skin on his belly button. Is that normal?

A: Your grandson may have a fairly common condition found in newborns (usually within the first few weeks of life) called an *umbilical granuloma*. The pinkish protrusion is actually scar tissue that didn't completely heal after the umbilical cord fell off. As the name implies, granulomas tend to have a grainy or crumbly texture. They also tend to produce sticky fluid. Unlike umbilical hernias, they're not covered with skin.

Why some babies get umbilical granulomas isn't clear, but it's not typically due to poor care (as some people might think). The granulomas usually disappear on their own in a week or so, but they may last for as long as a few months. Persistent granulomas or those that become irritated may require treatment, usually with silver nitrate. Very large ones may need to be removed.

If the tissue is a bright red, it could signal a much rarer and more serious congenital condition called an *umbilical polyp*. These polyps are actually remnants of intestinal, urinary tract, or other tissue. Unlike umbilical granulomas, they don't respond to treatment with silver nitrate. To prevent infec-

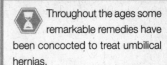

SIGNS OF THE TIMES

Throughout the ages some remarkable remedies have been concocted to treat umbilical hernias.

- In ancient Rome, a green male lizard was coaxed to bite the belly button of the afflicted child while he or she slept. The ancient Romans also occasionally applied a paste of burnt snail's ashes, frankincense, and white grape juice to the hernia.

- A 17th-century British doctor prescribed placing cow's dung, which had been boiled in milk, on a baby's swollen navel.

- In parts of Europe and the United States, goose droppings mixed with lard was a remedy used well into the 20th century.

- A potentially dangerous treatment that's still occasionally used today involves taping a coin over the baby's bulging belly button.

SIGNIFICANT FACT

"Innie" belly buttons are more common than "outie" ones. Some think that outies are caused by a tiny abdominal wall defect and others claim that the difference between innies and outies lies solely in how the umbilical cord was tied off.

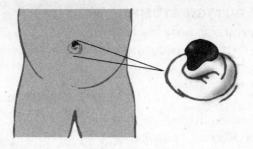

UMBILICAL GRANULOMA

tions or other serious complications, they may need to be surgically removed.

BABY LIMBS

LIMBER LIMBS

Q: *Our toddler is very double-jointed. He gets great pleasure from bending his fingers, arms, and legs in unusual positions. Can this be harmful?*

A: All babies are born "double-jointed." This doesn't mean that they literally have double joints; it means their joints are highly flexible. As they grow older, most children become less flexible, although as many as 20% remain very loose-jointed. Double-jointedness—medically referred to as *hypermobility, hyperflexibility,* or *laxity*—is usually a harmless condition. It often runs in families and tends to affect girls more than boys. Children who are hypermobile often have flat feet (see **Flat Feet,** below).

While it may scare parents to watch their child bend him- or herself into a pretzel, it's usually a safe practice when done in moderation. However, some children with hypermobile joints will suffer from joint pain, dislocations, muscle or tendon problems, or injuries. Special exercises are often recommended for these children to keep their muscles strong.

In rare cases, laxity may be a sign of the genetic connective-tissue disorder Marfan syndrome (see **Sunken Chest,** above). People with this uncommon condition tend to be very tall and thin and have long fingers and other extremities. (Abraham Lincoln is said to have had this condition.) They may also have funnel or pigeon chest. (See **Sunken Chest** and **Pointy Chest,** above.) It's important that Marfan be diagnosed early, because it's a progressive disorder that can lead to potentially serious eye, heart, lung, and other medical problems.

If your child has hypermobile joints as well as loose, stretchy skin that bruises easily, it may signal another rare, serious, genetic connective-tissue disorder called *Ehlers-Danlos syndrome*. There are several forms of this disorder that can range from mild to life threatening. Treatment depends on the specific effects and severity of the condition and can include exercise, physical therapy, injury prevention, and occasionally surgery.

BENT THUMB

Q: We've noticed recently that our 5-month-old son's right thumb is bent forward. It doesn't seem to hurt him, so we don't think it's broken. What else could be causing this?

A: It sounds as if your son has what's referred to as *congenital trigger thumb,* or more aptly, *pediatric trigger thumb* (rarely seen at birth, it usually shows up when a child is about 1 year of age). This is a condition in which the thumb becomes locked in a fixed position. When it affects any of the other fingers, it's called *trigger finger,* which is more common in adults.

Trigger thumb is usually painless and can affect one or both thumbs. In some cases, there's a bump or a nodule at the base of the thumb. The cause of trigger thumb is unknown, but it does run in some families.

In up to 60% of cases, a child's trigger thumb will spontaneously return to normal by the age of 2. If not, surgery may be required for the child to regain full use of his or her hand.

BOWED LEGS

Q: Our 14-month-old toddler looks very bowlegged. Should we worry?

A: It may surprise you to hear that *all* babies are born bowlegged! This happens because babies' legs are folded while they're in their mothers' wombs. The bowing may not become noticeable, however, until they first begin walking. Babies' legs usually start to straighten out in the second year of life. So for toddlers like your daughter, legs that bow out are probably not a cause for concern.

If a child's legs remain bent after about 3 years of age, however, he or she is considered to have *bowlegs,* medically called *genu varum*. This condition can be a warning sign of *rickets,* a bone disease that's caused by a vitamin D deficiency and is characterized by weak bones. Children between 6 and 24 months of age are at greatest risk for this disease, which can lead to severe muscle, limb, and back pain, or even bone fractures. To prevent a baby or toddler from getting rickets, make sure that he or she gets adequate amounts of vitamin D through food, sun exposure, or supplements. Less commonly, bowlegs can be an important warning sign of an excess intake of fluoride (see Chapter 6) or even lead poisoning.

WARNING SIGN

Although breast-feeding is the ideal form of nutrition for infants, it doesn't supply any vitamin D, which is necessary for preventing rickets. All breast-fed babies, therefore, require vitamin D supplements. The American Academy of Pediatrics increased their recommendation from 200 IU of vitamin D per day to 400 IU (for breast-fed babies, from birth).

Dark-skinned babies are at an especially increased risk for rickets because the *melanin* (dark pigment) in their skin can prevent absorption of vitamin D from the sun.

Bowlegs sometimes signal *Blount's disease* (aka *tibia vara*), a growth disorder of the shinbone that results in the severe bowing of one or both legs. It's usually first noticed in children between the ages of 2 and 4 years. It sometimes runs in families, and it affects more girls than boys. Early walkers, children of African descent, and obese babies are at increased risk for this progressive disease. Leg braces are usually successful in treating young children with Blount's, but surgery may sometimes be needed for adolescents.

Finally, bowing of the legs in any direction can be an early warning sign of a very rare genetic disorder called *osteogenesis imperfecta* or *brittle bone disease*. Signs of brittle bone disease include frequent fractures, short stature, discolored teeth (see Chapter 6), and a blue or gray tint to the whites (*sclera*) of a baby's eyes. As the name implies, children born with brittle bone disease have extremely fragile, easily breakable bones. Although there's no cure, many treatments are available to reduce fractures and pain.

KNOCK-KNEE

Q: *When our toddler toddles, his knees point inward. Will he outgrow it?*

A: Your son probably has what's commonly called *knock-knee* and medically known as *genu valgum*. As part of normal development, a toddler's knees often start to turn inward to help him or her maintain balance when walking. Indeed, most children become knock-kneed by the time they're 3 years old, and many remain that way until they're about 5 or 6 years of age. As with bowlegs (see **Bowed Legs,** above), overweight children are at increased risk for persistent knock-knee because their growing bones deform under their excess weight.

Besides being a cosmetic problem, persistent knock-knee can interfere with running and other physical activities. Physical therapy and

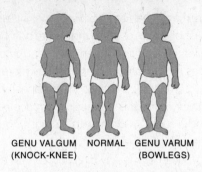

GENU VALGUM   NORMAL   GENU VARUM
(KNOCK-KNEE)   (BOWLEGS)

NORMAL AND ABNORMAL LEG ALIGNMENTS

braces are rarely helpful, and in extreme cases, surgery may be recommended.

Knock-knee that persists can also be a sign of an injury to the shinbone, an infection of the bone or bone marrow, or an underlying bone disease such as rickets (see **Bowed Legs,** above). These, however, would also involve more worrisome signs such as swelling, pain, and fever.

PIGEON TOES

Q: Our adopted daughter just started walking. Her feet turn inward and she trips a lot. Should we be concerned?

A: Toddlers often walk with their feet turned inward—medically called *intoeing* (aka *pigeon toes*). In most cases, this is the normal result of having spent 9 months in the fetal position. Whether present at birth or developed later, intoeing is typically a painless, benign condition. However, it may cause children like your daughter to have an increased tendency to trip and fall. The good news is that most children with this condition will soon

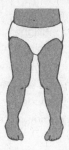

INTOEING (PIGEON-TOES)

learn to walk without tripping and will totally outgrow intoeing in a few years.

Most pigeon-toed children don't need any treatment because their feet will ultimately straighten out. In rare cases, however, intoeing may affect one foot more than the other, or the condition may worsen. If either of these things happens, further medical evaluation is needed. Physical therapy or other treatment may be necessary, but surgery is rarely required.

DUCK WALKING

Q: *Our 2-year-old son walks like a duck, with his feet pointing outward. Might there be something wrong with his feet?*

A: Walking with feet turned outward, called *out-toeing,* is less common than intoeing, but the causes are similar (see **Pigeon Toes,** above). Children with out-toeing often have flat feet (see **Flat Feet,** below). They may be late walkers, and once they start walking their out-turned feet may make them look unstable. Out-toeing sometimes runs in families, and it is more commonly seen in children who are heavier than normal. Like intoeing, out-toeing is not painful, and it normally resolves in a few years. Treatment is rarely required, except in extreme cases.

If, however, your son also waddles from side to side and/or limps, he may be showing signs of *developmental dysplasia of the hip (DDH)*, aka *congenital hip dysplasia,* a condition in which one or both of a baby's hips are dislocated or "out of joint." Although newborns are usually screened for this disorder, it's not always evident until a baby starts walking. Other signs include one leg that's shorter than the other, uneven or asymmetric skin folds on the thighs or buttocks, or a back that abnormally curves inward, commonly referred to as *swayback* and medically known as *lordosis.*

Although its cause is unknown, DDH tends to run in families and is much more common in girls, firstborn children, and breech babies. Babies who are swaddled are also at increased risk. (See **Swaddling,** below.)

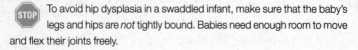

STOP SIGN

STOP　To avoid hip dysplasia in a swaddled infant, make sure that the baby's legs and hips are *not* tightly bound. Babies need enough room to move and flex their joints freely.

Early diagnosis and treatment are essential. If left untreated, hip dysplasia will lead to hip arthritis in early adulthood, which can be extremely painful and severely debilitating. Treatment usually involves braces or casts, and in severe cases surgery.

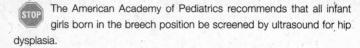

STOP SIGN

STOP　The American Academy of Pediatrics recommends that all infant girls born in the breech position be screened by ultrasound for hip dysplasia.

WALKING ON TIPPY TOES

Q: *Our little girl often walks on her tippy toes like a ballerina. While it looks cute, we wonder if something is wrong with her feet.*

A: Most toddlers will occasionally walk on their tiptoes. Usually there's no underlying muscle problem and the cause is unknown. Toe walking very rarely warrants concern—children who do it typically walk normally by the time they're 2 years old.

However, if a child *always* walks on tiptoes or will not stand with his or her heels on the floor, it may be a warning sign of an underlying problem, such as hip dysplasia. (See **Duck Walking,** above.) Another warning sign is if the child continues this behavior past the age of 2.

In rare cases toe walking could also signal a mild form of *cerebral palsy* (*CP*), a neuromuscular disorder. Other signs of mild CP may include lack of coordination, clumsiness, and such developmental delays as late walking and talking. Early treatment, which often involves braces and physical therapy, can improve a child's physical functioning as well as his or her self-esteem.

FLAT FEET

Q: *My 16-month-old son has flat feet. So do I. Did he inherit this from me and can something be done about it?*

A: Flat feet, medically known as *pronation* or *pes planus,* are exceedingly common in infants and toddlers. This is because the arches of a baby's foot take several years to fully develop. Most children with flat feet will have normal arches between the ages of 3 and 10.

However, flat feet, or fallen arches as they're also called, do often run in families, so it is possible that your son inherited them from you. They are also more common in children who have hypermobile joints. (See **Limber Limbs,** above.)

Because flat feet don't usually cause pain or other problems in babies and toddlers, treatment is rarely necessary. But if your son's feet are

SIGN OF THE TIMES

Most people's big toes—aka "great toes"—are longer than their second toes. This digit development is referred to as an *Egyptian foot,* named for how feet were depicted in ancient Egyptian art. When the second toe is the longer one, it's referred to as a *Greek* or *Grecian foot* because of the way ancient Greeks portrayed most feet. They believed that this toe formation, now medically known as *Morton's toe,* was a sign of good breeding. About 10% of people have this inherited trait.

flat and also seem stiff and inflexible, it may be due to *tarsal coalition*. This is a congenital and often inherited condition in which some bones in the foot fuse together. Although present at birth, tarsal coalition may go undiagnosed until adolescence. Anti-inflammatory drugs and other painkillers, physical therapy, and orthotics are used to treat this condition. In severe cases, surgery may be recommended.

OTHER TORSO TOPICS

SHUDDERING SPELLS

Q: Our 18-month-old daughter occasionally shudders quite severely. We were assured by our pediatrician that she's not having seizures, but we're still worried. Should we be?

A: It sounds as if your daughter has a fairly rare condition referred to as *shuddering attacks* (aka *benign paroxysmal spells of childhood*). These attacks typically last from about 5 to 15 seconds and may occur infrequently or up to several times a day. During an attack, the child's upper body or arms may shiver uncontrollably, and his or her body may stiffen. Shuddering attacks sometimes resemble mild epileptic seizures, for which they might be mistaken. But unlike epileptic seizures, they do not cause a child to lose consciousness. And while epileptic seizures may occur during sleep, shuddering attacks don't.

The cause of shuddering attacks is unknown, but they tend to run in families with a history of *essential tremors*. (See Chapter 6.) As scary as these attacks may appear, they're usually totally benign and most children outgrow them. Treatment is rarely necessary.

SWADDLING

Q: My mother-in-law suggested that swaddling would help calm my fussy newborn daughter. But one of my friends warned me that swaddling can harm a baby. Whom should I believe?

A: They're both right, to some extent. Since prehistoric times swaddling has been used to calm infants, straighten their limbs, and even prevent hernias (see **Belly Button Bulge,** above). In many cases, babies were very tightly bound and/or immobilized for long periods of time. Excessive swaddling fell out of favor in the mid-18th century when doctors and philosophers seriously clamped down on it, claiming that it was a harmful practice.

Today, swaddling has made a comeback in Europe and the United States. Most recent studies have confirmed that when done correctly, swaddling is often helpful in decreasing excessive crying and in promoting and prolonging sleep in newborns. And swaddling has also been found useful in reducing pain in infants who have to undergo blood tests and other painful procedures.

However, some recent studies have found that when done incorrectly, swaddling can increase the risk of developmental hip dysplasia (see **Duck Walking,** above), as well as hyperthermia (overheating). Finally, sleeping prone (on the stomach) while swaddled puts an infant at increased risk for sudden infant death syndrome (SIDS). Therefore, babies who are able to turn over on their stomachs by themselves

SIGN OF THE TIMES

One of the strangest uses of swaddling is to keep infants motionless during the Baby Jumping Festival. In this bizarre event—which is held annually in Castillo de Murcia in northern Spain—swaddled newborns are placed on the ground on mattresses. Dressed as devils, local men then leap over double rows of babies, much to the delight of the spectators, if not the parents and the babies themselves. This quasi-religious ceremony, which was first held in the 1620s, supposedly protects the infants by cleansing them of all evil.

SIGN OF THE TIMES

In parts of Europe and the United States, during the 18th century, swaddled babies were often hung from hooks on household walls or from trees in the field while their busy mothers or caregivers were working. This problematic practice purportedly kept the infants safe from household hazards and wild animals.

should no longer be swaddled. If you are interested in swaddling, be sure to discuss it with your baby's doctor. He or she can help you with your decision and teach you the safest technique.

SIGNING OFF

At birth, a baby's torso, arms, legs, fingers, and toes are all carefully examined. Physical abnormalities or other potential problems are usually detected at that point or soon afterward at well-baby check-ups. But many torso- and limb-related conditions can crop up at any point during infancy and toddlerhood. And parents are often the first to notice the significant signs.

CALL YOUR BABY'S DOCTOR AS SOON AS POSSIBLE
IF YOUR BABY HAS:

- Bloody or foul-smelling discharge or pus coming from a nipple
- Chills that cause him or her to shake all over
- Recently started limping
- Difficulty moving an arm, leg, finger, or toes
- Swelling or prolonged pain after injury to any part of the body
- An arm, leg, hand, or foot that suddenly seems stuck in one position or bent out of shape

CALL YOUR BABY'S DOCTOR OR 911 IMMEDIATELY
IF YOUR BABY HAS:

- Bloody or foul-smelling discharge or pus coming from the navel
- Difficulty moving his or her head
- A stiff neck with a high fever
- Convulsions, seizures, or other uncontrollable movements
- Sudden weakness or paralysis in any part of his or her body
- Prolonged bleeding from any part of the body

CHAPTER 8

YOUR BABY'S SKIN

There's not a rose where'er I seek
As comely as my baby's cheek.
    —Anonymous, "Mother's Song"

SKIN IS OUR LARGEST ORGAN, and it's the only one that's entirely on the outside of our bodies. As a result, it's exposed to endless irritants, starting even in the womb. For example, a fetus's skin is constantly bathed in amniotic fluid, which is primarily composed of the fetus's own urine. But a fetus's skin is quite resilient; it's protected by a thick, white, waxy coating called *vernix* and fine hairs called *lanugo*. Much to the surprise and dismay of many new parents, newborns are usually coated with vernix at birth. And some have lanugo on their face, trunk, or limbs. The good news is that the vernix usually washes off during the baby's first bath, and the lanugo disappears within the first few weeks.

A newborn's skin color may be different from what his or her parents expect. Regardless of a baby's race, the typical healthy newborn's skin color will range from dark red to purple at birth. Over the next few days, the infant's skin will go through several color changes. It can

SIGNIFICANT FACTS

⚠ Babies born prematurely are more likely to have lanugo than those who are born full-term. Their skin is also thinner and more transparent, making their veins more visible.

take up to 6 months for the baby's skin to take on its permanent color.

And then there are the infamous birthmarks—so common in newborns, yet so frequently unwelcome by their parents. New moms and dads may dislike the appearance of these discolorations—which can sometimes be quite large and unattractive—and fear that they'll never go away. They may even worry that they're a sign of something that's wrong with their baby.

Because a newborn's skin is so visible, new parents tend to focus, sometimes excessively or obsessively, on it. And some skin signs do, in fact, warrant special attention from parents and physicians. For example, many allergies, infections, hormonal imbalances, systemic diseases, and even signs of physical abuse are often first spotted on the skin. Happily, most birthmarks, rashes, and other skin problems seen on newborns, infants, and toddlers are usually nothing to worry about, and often disappear on their own. But because it's not always easy to distinguish between the benign and potentially bad skin signs, they should all be mentioned to and carefully evaluated by the baby's doctor.

BIRTHMARKS

RED OR PINK BIRTHMARK

Q: *Our twins were born with red birthmarks; our daughter has one on her face and our son's is on his neck. What caused them and will they ever go away?*

A: It sounds like your twins have the most common type of *vascular birthmark,* called a *macular (flat) stain.* Also known as *nevus simplex* or *salmon patches,* they're found on up to 50%

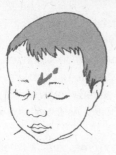

ANGEL KISS

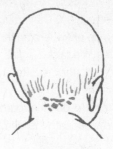

STORK BITE

of babies at or shortly after birth. They're neither inherited nor caused by anything that might have happened during pregnancy. Rather, they're the result of dilation or an increased number of blood vessels, which occur for unknown reasons.

These birthmarks are usually flat and red or pink. They may fade when pressed on and darken when the baby cries. They can be found on any part of the body but are usually spotted on the neck or face, especially on the eyelids, nose, lips, or forehead. When they're in these locations, they're called "angel kisses." The good news is that angel

kisses usually disappear by the time the child is 2 years old. When the marks show up on the back of a baby's neck, however, they're called stork bites and they tend to be permanent.

LARGE, LUMPY BIRTHMARK

Q: *My 1-month-old grandson has a large, ugly, reddish mark on his arm. I notice that it keeps getting bigger. My daughter-in-law says it's a "strawberry birthmark" and nothing to worry about. Is she right?*

A: Your daughter-in-law is probably referring to a common type of vascular birthmark (see **Red or Pink Birthmark,** above) called an *infantile hemangioma*. Hemangiomas are noncancerous lesions composed of dense masses of dilated blood vessels, which often show up a few weeks after birth. They're usually found on the head and neck, but they can pop up anywhere on the body. In most cases, a baby has only one, which may be raised or flat. Because these birthmarks tend to look like ripened fruit, they're often referred to as *strawberry* or *cherry hemangiomas*. There's another type called *deep* or *cavernous hemangiomas,* which tend to be blue, purple, or flesh-colored. As their name implies, they grow beneath the skin.

Hemangiomas are 3 times more common in girls than in boys and much more common in white babies than in black or Asian babies. Indeed, about 1 in 10 white infants have them. The cause of hemangiomas, like other birthmarks, is unknown. However, pre-term and low-birth-weight babies are at an increased risk.

Hemangiomas usually grow rapidly during a baby's 1st year or so. They may reach 2 inches in diameter or larger and can be quite unsightly, especially when they're on a baby's face. The good news is that when a child is about a year old, most hemangiomas stop growing, lighten, and slowly begin to shrink. And by the time a child is 9 years old, the vast majority of these birthmarks will have disappeared or flattened and faded, becoming much less noticeable.

SIGN OF THE TIMES

Over the past 20 years, the incidence of hemangiomas in infants has risen an estimated 40%. Researchers believe this is due to the increase in low-birth-weight babies, perhaps as a result of infertility treatments and advanced maternal age. Hemangiomas are also seen more often in babies whose mothers have undergone a prenatal test called *chorionic villus sampling.*

Because most hemangiomas are only of cosmetic concern and are likely to disappear, treatment usually isn't necessary. However, some may ulcerate, bleed, and become infected, in which case they may need to be surgically removed. In rare cases, a hemangioma can impinge on an organ and cause potentially serious problems. For example, if it's on the head or neck, a baby's vision, hearing, breathing, or eating can be affected. Hemangiomas on the lower back may be related to spinal problems, and those on the genitals may be associated with urinary and pelvic disorders. Therefore, careful monitoring is necessary and surgical removal may be required.

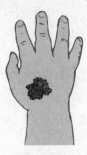

HEMANGIOMA

BURGUNDY BIRTHMARK

Q: *Our infant son has a rather large dark red birthmark over his eye. Will it affect his vision?*

A: It sounds like your son has a *port-wine stain,* medically known as *nevus flammeus.* These birthmarks, which are usually flat with irregular borders, are most often seen on the face, but they may also be found on the trunk, arms, or legs. Although they may not be visible immediately, they are present at birth. Like salmon patches (see **Red or Pink Birthmarks,** above), port-wine stains are vascular birthmarks. But unlike salmon patches,

they're not very common, and they tend to grow and thicken over time.

Depending on their location, port-wine stains, which are permanent, are usually only a cosmetic concern and nothing to worry about medically. However, children who have one of these birthmarks over an eye

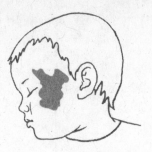

PORT-WINE STAIN

may be at increased risk for glaucoma and other vision problems and should be carefully watched. Port-wine stains on the legs may increase the risk of varicose veins and, in very rare cases, bone growth disorders.

Port-wine stains on a baby's upper eyelid and forehead can be the earliest signs of a very rare congenital neurological disorder, *Sturge-Weber syndrome*. Children with this disorder, which is not hereditary, usually have seizures by the time they're a year old and may develop other neurological conditions and eye disorders, especially glaucoma. Although there is no cure for Sturge-Weber, the convulsions and other complications it causes can be treated with medication and sometimes surgery.

BLUE BIRTHMARK

Q: My infant niece has a blue patch near her eye. My brother says it's just a birthmark, but I thought birthmarks were red. Are blue ones different?

A: Although most birthmarks are reddish, they can come in a variety of colors, including blue. If a birthmark is lumpy as well as blue, it may be a deep hemangioma (see **Large, Lumpy Birthmark,** above). If, however, the mark is speckled and flat, and your niece is of Asian descent, she may have a condition called *nevus of Ota*. These patches, which are mostly seen on Japanese children, are usually blue or gray and commonly appear on the face. Sometimes the whites of the baby's eyes (*sclera*) will also have a blue tint.

Genes often play a key role in causing these birthmarks. Hormones may be linked to them as well; the patches tend to darken with age, especially during puberty. Although usually just a cosmetic concern, a nevus over the eye may signal an increased risk of glaucoma. And in very rare cases a nevus can be a warning sign of potential *melanoma* (the deadliest skin cancer). So though these marks are often harmless, they should be carefully monitored.

BLACK-AND-BLUE BIRTHMARKS

Q: *Our baby was born with what looks like bruises on his legs. Can they be from childbirth and will they go away?*

A: Some babies are, in fact, born with bruises. They're usually found on the face or scalp, and result from a difficult and/or forceps delivery. Such bruises often disappear in a few days. But blue marks that don't soon disappear are more likely a common type of pigmented birthmark called *Mongolian spots*. These spots, which can be blue or grayish, are most often seen on dark-skinned children. Indeed, up to 90% of children of Native American, African, Hispanic, and Asian descent have at least one of them.

Mongolian spots are typically found on the lower back, buttocks, legs, and sometimes arms. They're usually round or oval and measure about ½ inch to 2 inches, but some are much bigger. A baby can be born with one or more of them. Because of their location and color, Mongolian spots are often mistaken for bruises. But unlike black-and-blue marks, which change color and fade rather quickly, these marks don't.

WARNING SIGN

Because Mongolian spots look like bruises and are on parts of the body where abused children are often struck, they are sometimes mistaken for signs of abuse. In fact, many parents of babies with these birthmarks have been falsely accused of child abuse. Therefore, it's important for parents of babies with Mongolian spots to tell day-care and school officials about these marks and their locations.

Mongolian spots are totally benign, requiring no treatment. In most children they disappear completely within a few years, but in some they are permanent.

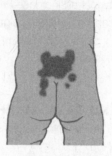

MONGOLIAN SPOTS

FRECKLES

LOTS OF FRECKLES

Q: *I thought that only blondes and redheads get freckles. But our dark-haired, dark-skinned toddler has lots of them. What could be the cause?*

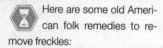

A: Freckles are usually an inherited trait in families with blond or red hair and fair skin, but they can appear in children with dark hair and skin as well. Medically known as *ephelides,* freckles are actually clusters of concentrated *melanin,* the pigment that gives skin, hair, and eyes their color.

Freckles are not present at birth. Rather, they tend to show up at around 2 years of age from sun exposure. They're usually small and flat, and they typically occur in clusters on sun-exposed areas such as the nose, cheeks, shoulders, and back. The more sun exposure, the darker and more noticeable they become. Indeed, an abundance of freckles on a baby or child is an important warning sign that they've been out in the sun too much and are at an increased risk for developing skin cancer.

Freckled babies who are *extremely* sensitive to the sun, especially if they have dark skin, may have a very rare genetic condition called *xeroderma pigmentosum* (*XP*). These babies may have extremely light-sensitive eyes as well. In most cases the earliest sign of this disorder is a severe burn the first time a baby is exposed to the sun. Children with XP are at risk for serious eye and skin diseases, including skin cancer, which will often develop during early childhood. Because there's no cure for this condition, total protection from the sun is essential. Certain medications can also help protect the child from severe sunburns.

When freckles appear in skin folds and areas not normally exposed to the sun, such as the armpit, groin, and even on the palms, they may be a sign of *neurofibromatosis,* another rare genetic disease that varies in severity. When this potentially disfiguring condition occurs in infancy, it can cause skin tumors and deformed bones, and can also affect the skin, eyes, ears, bones, brain, blood vessels, heart, kidneys, and other internal organs. Although there is no cure, medication, radiation, and surgery can often help relieve the complications of neurofibromatosis.

STOP SIGN

 Just one blistering sunburn in childhood doubles the risk of the deadliest skin cancer, melanoma, later in life. To reduce the risk of skin cancer, all babies and toddlers should avoid exposure to direct sunlight. This is especially important for those with moles and/or fair skin.

LARGE FRECKLES

Q: Our daughter has several large freckles on her back. The pediatrician says they're "café au lait" spots and are nothing to worry about. But a woman in my new mothers' group told me that these spots can be a sign of a tumor. Is she right?

A: Café au lait spots are quite common and are usually nothing to worry about. These flat, discolored spots (aka *macules*) can range in color

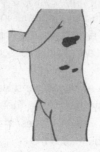

CAFÉ AU LAIT SPOTS

from light tan to dark brown. (In fact, *café au lait* is the French term for "coffee with milk.") They usually appear by the time a child is 3 years old, and they can occur anywhere on the body. They are more common in babies of African and Hispanic descent than in white babies.

Having a few café au lait spots, as your daughter does, is usually of no concern. But if a baby has 6 or more large spots (over ½ inch in diameter), it can be a warning sign of several rare, serious genetic disorders. These include *neurofibromatosis,* which can cause tumors in various parts of the body (see **Lots of Freckles,** above) and *McCune-Albright syndrome*, which affects the bones, skin, and endocrine system. Although there is no cure for either condition, medical treatments may help reduce or alleviate some of their symptoms.

LIP FRECKLES

Q: *My 16-month-old godson has dark freckles around his lips. Neither of his parents has freckles. I heard that this can be a sign of a serious condition. Could it be?*

A: While most freckles are inherited, anyone can develop them. (See **Lots of Freckles,** above.) They usually appear on sun-exposed areas of the skin and are almost always unrelated to disease.

Dark freckles on or around an infant's lips can be totally benign. But they can also be one of the earliest warning signs of a serious but very rare genetic disease, *Peutz-Jeghers syndrome* (*PJS*). The earliest signs of this condition are freckles inside a newborn's mouth, which may go unnoticed. By the time they're 2 years old, though, babies with PJS

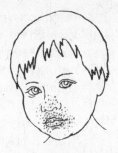

PEUTZ-JEGHERS SYNDROME

commonly have freckles on their lips, cheeks, nose, or hands. These freckles may be brown, black, or blue. As the children grow older, freckles may also show up on skin that's not normally exposed to the sun, such as the palms, soles, anus, or genitals.

Although the freckles themselves are harmless and will often fade or even disappear during puberty, PJS can lead to serious intestinal problems. These include polyps and obstructions in children (and adults). For this reason, PJS is also known as *hereditary intestinal polyposis syndrome*. Because the polyps often don't occur until a child is around 10 years old, PJS typically goes undiagnosed for years. Indeed, it may not be recognized until the polyps or obstruction cause pain or other problems, which usually occurs when people with this condition are in their 20s.

PJS can lead to colon cancer in adulthood, and it also increases the risk of gastrointestinal, breast, cervical, ovarian, pancreatic, and other cancers in later life. The good news is that removal of polyps or other growths can help prevent many of these cancers.

PIMPLES AND BLISTERS

BABY BLEMISHES

Q: We've just brought our first baby home and she has tiny bumps on her face. What could they be?

A: It sounds like your new daughter has the very common and normal skin condition called *milia*. Milia are small, white or pearly, pinpoint

A small, white or yellow, solid, round pimple on the heel of a newborn may be a *calcinosis cutis,* a telltale sign that a baby has had one or more blood samples taken from a heel stick. These pimples usually resolve on their own.

raised spots (*papules*) that are usually found on the nose, cheeks, and forehead of newborns a day or two after birth. Sometimes, however, they don't show up for a couple of weeks.

Milia are filled with fatty secretions and a waxy protein called *keratin*. These pimplelike bumps are similar to *Epstein's pearls,* which are commonly seen in the mouths of newborns. (See Chapter 6.) Because milia typically disappear within a few weeks after birth no treatment is required.

BABY ACNE

Q: We're expecting our first child. A friend told us that babies can get acne. Is this true? I had acne as a teenager and am really concerned.

A: There are 2 very common and inconsequential pimplelike conditions seen in babies. One is milia (see **Baby Blemishes,** above) and the other is *neonatal* or *baby acne*. Baby acne is more noticeable than milia, and its bumps show up a few days *after* birth rather than *at* birth. Baby acne is thought to be caused by some of the hormones that pass from mother to baby in the womb.

Neonatal acne looks much like the acne of puberty—little bumps or *pustule*s (small collections of pus) that may have whiteheads or blackheads in the center. These tiny pimples or red bumps can pop up on a baby's nose, cheeks, forehead, and scalp. In general, baby acne is nothing to worry about. It usually goes away quickly—although in some cases it may last for several months.

There's another slightly more serious and persistent type of acne that affects some babies, called *infantile acne* or *acne neonatorum*. Unlike the more common neonatal acne, this type of acne shows up when a baby is around 3 months of age or older. And infantile acne can last longer, sometimes until a child is 3 years old. It's more common in boys than in girls and is thought to be hormone-related. There may also be a genetic component because it's sometimes seen in children whose parents had acne during their teenage years. In mild cases no treatment is needed, but in more severe ones, permanent scarring may occur and topical agents and antibiotics might be necessary. Babies with infantile acne are also at increased risk for developing acne during puberty.

STOP SIGN

STOP   There's been a recent outbreak of rashes on the bodies of babies who've worn clothes made in China. The clothing was found to have high levels of formaldehyde—up to 900 times the normal limit. Regardless of where they're made, all new baby clothes, sheets, and towels should be carefully washed before being worn.

BABY BLISTERS

Q: *Our newborn daughter has yellowish blisters on her chest. Is this something she could have picked up in the hospital?*

A: Small yellow or white blisterlike bumps on a newborn may be a very common, noncontagious, and harmless skin condition with a rather scary name—*erythema toxicum neonatorum* (*ETN*). As many as 70% of full-term infants, especially those whose birth weight is above average, develop these skin eruptions, usually within the first 2 weeks after birth. ETN is more common in boys than in girls.

These skin bumps are usually surrounded by red, inflamed areas. They resemble fleabites, and like fleabites, they can number in the dozens. Some people mistakenly think they're hives.

ETN are most commonly found on the chest and back but sometimes show up on the face, arms, and legs as well. They're almost never seen on the palms of the hands and soles of the feet, which helps differentiate ETN from similar-looking skin conditions.

The cause of these unsightly eruptions is unclear, but some think that

SPEAKING OF SIGNS

A child about three days after delivery struck out all over the body with small red eruptions; which in London the nurses call the red-gum, but in Scotland is named the hives.

—Description of erythema toxicum neonatorum (ETN) from an 18th-century midwifery textbook the immune system may play a role. ETN usually resolves on its own within 2 weeks, but it can sometimes last as long as 6 weeks. Once these bumps disappear, they seldom return.

HONEYCOMB-LIKE BLISTERS

Q: *I was told that a toddler in my son's play group has impetigo and that it's very contagious. What else should I know about it?*

A: *Impetigo* is a bacterial skin infection that is, indeed, highly contagious. Your son's friend, and even his toys and security blanket, could quickly spread his infection to others. Impetigo is typically caused by staph or strep bacteria, and it affects mainly 2- to 6-year-olds—children at increased risk because their immune systems aren't mature enough to fight off these common germs.

About 70% of cases of impetigo start out as tiny blisters that break, ooze a thin, amber-colored fluid, and dry, leaving a characteristic honeycomb-like crust. Typically, these crusts are seen on the face, nose, and/or mouth, but sometimes they also appear on the neck, hands, and diaper area. About 30% of cases cause large blisters, which tend not to ooze.

Because impetigo is often itchy, scratching can break the blisters and spread the infection to other parts of the body. Keeping children from scratching and teaching them good hygiene can keep impetigo from infecting other areas of their bodies as well as other family members and friends. Opinion is mixed on how long impetigo stays contagious, but most experts agree that it's usually noncontagious within a

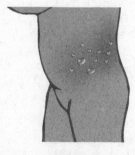

IMPETIGO

couple of days of starting treatment, which typically involves topical and/or oral antibiotics.

TRAVELING DIAPER RASH

Q: *The skin around our 18-month-old son's groin is red and peeling. We thought it was diaper rash, but now it's around his neck. Could it be something else?*

A: Distinguishing between the many common rashes that show up on babies can be difficult (particularly those that appear on the baby's bottom). A rash in the skin folds—such as the groin, neck, or underarms, and even between the toes and fingers—may be a condition called *intertrigo*. It's a type of skin inflammation (*dermatitis*) that occurs when skin chafes against skin, particularly when the skin is hot and sweaty. Other signs that a rash may be intertrigo are if it's a burnt-red color and it looks the same on both sides of a skin crease. Chubby babies are more likely to get this skin condition because their extra rolls of skin are ideal breeding grounds for bacteria.

Because a baby's skin is very delicate, intertrigo, like other types of diaper rash, can cause it to become red and irritated. As a result, babies with this condition are very prone to developing yeast, bacterial, or (in rare cases) viral infections. If there's no infection, simple measures such as keeping the skin clean and dry should help. If there is an infection, an antibiotic or antifungal may be needed.

BABY BUMPS AND LUMPS

HAIRY MOLES

Q: *Our 4-month-old daughter has several moles, including a few hairy ones. Is it normal for a baby to have moles, especially hairy ones?*

SIGNS OF THE TIMES

Since ancient Roman times, moles, especially on the cheeks, lips, and shoulders, have been seen as signs of beauty, hence the term "beauty marks." But moles on the nose have long been considered a no-no; they are associated with evil and witches. In China, nose moles are believed to be a harbinger of misfortune.

A: Many children have moles. In fact, about 1 in 100 newborns do. When moles are present at birth or appear a few days later, they're called *congenital nevi* or *congenital hairy nevi,* even though they don't always have hair growing from them in infancy. Coarse hairs will develop in some congenital moles, usually by the time a child is 2 years old.

Also known as *pigmented* or *melanocytic nevi,* moles often run in families. A child can have one or several moles, which can be light, dark, flat, or raised. They're usually round or oval with smooth edges.

Moles are sometimes mistaken for freckles. But unlike freckles, which aren't present at birth, moles often are. And while freckles show up on sun-exposed areas, moles can occur anywhere on the body, including between fingers and toes, in body folds, and on the genitals.

Most moles are less than ¼ inch in diameter (about the width of a pencil eraser) and are referred to as *small nevi*. In babies, moles that are larger than 4 inches are called *giant (hairy) nevi* and are very rare. (By adulthood, these moles usually grow to be 8 inches or more.) As children grow older, their moles can grow and darken.

Any type of congenital nevi can develop into skin cancer, including *melanoma,* the most deadly form. The larger the mole, the greater the risk of it becoming cancerous, even in babies. Also, the more moles a child (or adult) has, the higher the risk. Anyone with more than 50 moles is at especially high risk for melanoma. Sun exposure, even in moderate

WARNING SIGNS

Signs of possible skin cancer in a child (or an adult) include:
- A sudden increase in the size of a mole or birthmark
- Bleeding of a skin growth
- Inflamed or ulcerated skin growth
- Change in color of a mole or birthmark

amounts, significantly increases this risk. All congenital moles, regardless of their size, should be carefully monitored. In some cases, surgical removal is recommended.

SKIN TAG

Q: Our toddler has what looks like a skin tag on his neck. Do babies get skin tags?

A: Your baby probably has what's medically known as a *cutaneous cervical tag* or more commonly by the unattractive moniker, *wattle*, which is very rare. Wattles are flesh-colored bits of skin that usually pop out on or near the necks of children younger than 3 years of age. They're equally common in girls and in boys. Rarely, a child may have more than one tag; in these cases, the additional tags will likely occur on the opposite side of the neck from the original one.

Wattles are believed to be benign remnants from the fetal development of the ears and neck. In most cases, they're only a cosmetic concern and can easily be removed. In rare cases, they may be associated with an abnormality of the neck and may require more extensive surgery.

ORANGE BUMP ON THE FACE

Q: My baby girl has a little orange bump on her eyelid. What could it be?

A: Your daughter might have a rare skin condition, found primarily in infants, called *juvenile xanthogranuloma (JXG)*. Although rather scary-sounding, JXG is usually totally harmless. In most cases, only a single, firm orange or reddish-brown bump is seen on the face, especially around the eyes. Occasionally, however, these bumps may appear on other parts of the body.

JXG affects boys more frequently than girls, and it is 10 times more common in whites than in blacks. While it can be present at birth, it usually shows up sometime during the first year. Babies younger than 6 months of age who have JXG often have several bumps.

The good news is that this condition is usually benign and spontaneously disappears on its own. However, some children with juvenile xanthogranuloma also have café au lait spots. (See **Large Freckles,** above.) Children who have both of these skin conditions are at increased risk for epilepsy.

In rare cases, JXG can occur *inside* the eye and cause bleeding. Some of these *hyphemas,* as they're medically known, resolve on their own. Others may require treatment to help prevent vision problems, including possible loss of vision.

BABY DIMPLES

LEG DIMPLE

Q: *My newborn daughter has a large dimple on her leg. I thought dimples cropped up only on chins and cheeks. Is it possible that her skin dent isn't a dimple?*

A: While dimples are mostly found on a child's face, they can appear on any part of the baby's body. Dimples are usually an inherited trait, but a dimple on an infant can also be the result of a needle puncture during *amniocentesis*. If the needle happens to touch the growing fetus's delicate skin, it can leave an indentation, which may look like a dimple.

Amniocentesis-related dimples are not as common as they once were. Improvements in ultrasound guidance during the procedure have made it easier to avoid touching and puncturing the fetus's delicate skin. If these needle-related dimples do occur, they're permanent, but also totally benign.

BACK DIMPLE

Q: *My grandson has a dimple on his back, just above his buttocks. None of my 6 other grandchildren had anything like that, so I'm concerned. Should I be?*

A: Your grandson may have what's medically known as a *sacral* or *pilonidal dimple*. These are fairly common, occurring in about 4% of all babies. Sacral dimples are found at the base of the spine, just above the crease of the buttocks. Some are surrounded by hair and others may have hair growing inside them.

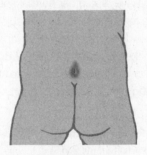

SACRAL DIMPLE

In most cases, sacral dimples are totally harmless and are not associated with any diseases or disorders. If, however, they're deep, they should be kept clean to avoid infections and cysts from forming. This tends to happen most often in older children, and when it does, surgery may be needed to drain the cyst.

In rare cases, a sacral dimple can be a sign of a mild form of *spina bifida* (SB), called *closed* or *hidden neural tube defect*. (SB is a birth defect in which the tissue surrounding the spinal cord fails to close during early gestation.) In these cases, the dimples tend to be larger, deeper, and farther away from the buttocks. A small tuft of hair may grow from inside the indentation, rather than surrounding the dimple.

Some children with closed neural tube defect may have few, if any, medical problems; others may have nerve damage, leg weakness or paralysis, and urinary or bowel problems. Medication, physical therapy, and sometimes surgery may help minimize these difficulties.

SKIN COLOR CHANGES

BLUE SKIN

Q: *I've been told that it's normal for babies to turn blue when they cry, but that they can turn blue when there's something medically wrong too. How can I tell the difference?*

A: It's true that when babies cry, the skin around their mouths will often take on a blue or purplish tinge, medically known as *cyanosis*. This is indeed quite normal, and the blue will go away when the baby calms down and stops crying. There are also other normal and benign reasons why babies might turn blue temporarily. Because babies are sensitive to temperature, their fingers and toes may become cyanotic when they're cold. A bruise can also turn the skin blue. (See **Easy Bruising,** below.)

But cyanosis can signal a myriad of moderate to serious medical conditions as well, including blood, metabolic, heart, and lung disorders.

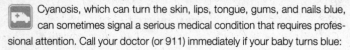

DANGER SIGN

Cyanosis, which can turn the skin, lips, tongue, gums, and nails blue, can sometimes signal a serious medical condition that requires professional attention. Call your doctor (or 911) immediately if your baby turns blue:

- For several minutes
- While resting
- While having difficulty breathing

YELLOW OR ORANGISH SKIN

Q: *We just adopted a baby girl, and her skin has a yellow cast to it. Could she have jaundice?*

A: Yellow skin is, indeed, a sign of jaundice. This is a very common and usually harmless condition in newborns, in which their skin, eyes, and sometimes stools take on a yellowish tinge (see Chapters 3 and 10). Jaundice is the result of a buildup of *bilirubin,* a yellow-orange substance produced by the breakdown of red blood cells in the liver.

Jaundice can sometimes signal various medical conditions ranging from mild to serious, especially if it persists after the newborn period or

first occurs after it. For example, mild
jaundice can be a sign of a benign,
hereditary condition called *Gilbert's
syndrome*. Gilbert's is quite common—about 3% to 5% of the general
population has it. With this syndrome,

jaundice tends to appear during times of exertion, stress, not eating,
and infection. Fortunately, it doesn't usually cause any health problems,
so no treatment is needed.

Very yellow or orange skin can signal dangerously high levels of
bilirubin, which can lead to such serious disorders as liver disease,
deafness, cerebral palsy, and even brain damage. Prompt treatment,
which may involve phototherapy and/or an exchange blood transfusion, can usually prevent these devastating consequences.

But yellow- or orange-tinged skin isn't only a sign of jaundice. It can
also be a telltale sign of *carotenemia,* a condition caused by an excess of
beta-carotene in the blood. The prime culprit for carotenemia is con-
sumption of a large amount of carrots, sweet potato, or pumpkin. Deep
green or yellow vegetables and fruits may also contain high levels of beta-
carotene. Even egg yolks and milk are rich in this important nutrient.

Carotenemia-caused yellow-orange skin is most visible in babies
and toddlers with light complexions. It's typically noticeable on the parts
of the body that tend to sweat, such as the palms, the soles of the feet,
and the skin around the nose and mouth. The discoloration is also more

visible in artificial light. Fortunately, carotenemia is harmless and usually goes away when a wider variety of foods is added to a baby's diet.

MARBLED SKIN

Q: *I was babysitting for my new niece and noticed some weblike marks under her skin. Is that normal?*

A: Your niece may have a common condition called *cutis marmorata,* which often occurs during a baby's first few months of life. The skin's marbled or mottled appearance is due largely to the immaturity of the blood vessels near the surface of the baby's skin. Some of these blood vessels constrict, giving the skin a bluish tint, and others dilate, giving it a reddish color. The result: a fishnetlike effect. The skin might look blotchier when the baby is cold, with the blotches fading when the baby warms up. Cutis marmorata is harmless and usually disappears as babies get a little older.

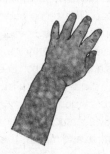

CUTIS MARMORATA (MOTTLED SKIN)

There's another extremely rare form of this condition called *cutis marmorata telangiectatica congenita (CMTC),* in which the skin color change tends to be more noticeable and is not likely to go away when the baby comes in from the cold. This condition is more common in children who live in cold climates.

Although CMTC is usually benign, about half of babies with it will also have other skin conditions, such as port-wine stains (see **Burgundy Birthmark,** above) and hemangiomas (see **Large, Lumpy Birthmark,** above). They are also at increased risk for bone, teeth, or eye problems. CMTC itself doesn't require treatment, and children who have it will usually outgrow it by the time they're teenagers, if not much sooner.

LIGHT SKIN PATCHES

Q: *A boy in my son's play group has large white patches on his arms. What could they be?*

A: Areas of white skin are a hallmark of *vitiligo*, a chronic skin condition characterized by patches that lack pigmentation. Some people confuse vitiligo with *albinism;* but albinism, which is a genetic disorder present from birth, is the complete or nearly complete absence of pigment in the eyes, hair, or skin. (See Chapters 2 and 3.)

Vitiligo is a benign, fairly common skin disorder that affects about 1 in 100 people of all ages. Although it usually first appears between the ages of 10 and 30, infants and babies can also get it. It occurs in all races but is more noticeable in people with dark skin. Although the cause is unknown, it's believed to be an autoimmune disorder. It sometimes runs in families.

Vitiligo patches, which sometimes get larger with time, typically show up on sun-exposed areas, especially the face, arms, and hands. But they can also occur in skin folds, around the genitals, and inside the nose and mouth.

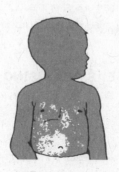

VITILIGO

Vitiligo occurs most often in people with such autoimmune diseases as *hyperthyroidism, alopecia areata* (see Chapter 2), and *pernicious anemia,* a blood disorder caused by inadequate vitamin B_{12}. Although there's no cure for vitiligo, treatments are available to fade the spots, help stop or delay their appearance, and even restore some skin color in the affected areas. Babies and toddlers are often treated with a topical corticosteroid, which is sometimes used with ultraviolet light treatment.

> **WARNING SIGN**
>
> Babies (and adults) with vitiligo need extra sun protection. The white patches it causes are highly susceptible to sunburn, and many of the treatments for it temporarily increase the risk of severe sunburn.

BABY BRUISES

BABY HICKEY

Q: My 3-month-old has what looks like a hickey on her arm. What could it be?

A: It sounds as if your baby may have a *suction blister.* These blisters are, in fact, similar to hickeys; they're the result of an infant sucking his or her arm, hand, fingers, or even toes. In fact, babies have been known to be born with these blisters on their extremities from vigorous sucking in the womb. Whether they occur prenatally or neonatally, they are usually nothing to worry about—they'll resolve on their own. But a cluster of blisters, particularly if they break open and leave behind a yellowish-brown crust, may signal the highly contagious skin infection impetigo, which requires treatment with antibiotics. (See **Honeycomb-Like Blisters,** above.)

EASY BRUISING

Q: Our toddler is very active and is always getting black-and-blue marks. My mother worries that he may have a blood disease such as leukemia. Could she be right?

A: Easy bruising can certainly result from rough-and-tumble play. In these cases, potential injuries are probably more of a concern than the bruises themselves. But frequent bruising can also signal a number of blood diseases, as your mother mentioned, as well as other medical disorders.

Babies who have *iron-deficiency anemia* tend to bruise easily. Other signs of this condition, which tends to affect babies between 9 and 24 months, include paleness, fatigue, irritability, swollen tongue, brittle nails, and loss of appetite. Low-birth-weight and premature babies are at increased risk for iron-deficiency anemia. Treatment is very simple and effective: iron-rich foods or iron supplements.

Easy bruising can also be a warning sign of *Ehlers-Danlos syndrome* (*EDS*), a group of rare genetic connective-tissue disorders. (Connective tissues hold the body structures together, including the ligaments, bone, cartilage, blood vessels, and organs.) Other common signs include loose joints (see Chapter 7) and easily stretchable skin. Some forms of EDS are very mild, while others are life threatening. Depending on the severity of the condition and the parts of the body affected, treatment may include exercise, physical therapy, injury prevention, and occasionally surgery.

A baby who bruises easily *and* has frequent broken bones may have another rare genetic disorder, *osteogenesis imperfecta,* aka *brittle bone disease* (see Chapters 1 and 7). Other signs may include loose joints, bowlegs or other bone deformities, and brittle or discolored teeth. Because of their broken bones, these children are often mistaken for being victims of child abuse. Although there's no cure for brittle bone disease, various treatments can help reduce fractures and other problems.

STOP SIGN

 To prevent iron-deficiency anemia, make sure babies who breast-feed after 4 months of age get iron through food or supplements. Infants who drink cow's milk or formula that doesn't contain iron also need iron from other sources.

Finally, as your mother mentioned, easy bruising does sometimes signal *leukemia,* a cancer of the white blood cells. Although it's the most common type of childhood cancer, it's still very rare. Other signs include easy bleeding (especially frequent nosebleeds), paleness, weakness, fatigue, loss of appetite, and persistent infections and fevers. A child with leukemia may also have a swollen belly or lymph nodes. White and

Hispanic children are at increased risk, and while leukemia sometimes runs in families, most cases are not inherited.

The good news is that with early diagnosis and treatment, the cure rate for childhood leukemia is extremely high, up to 85%. Treatments typically involve radiation and/or chemotherapy. In some cases, bone marrow and blood stem cell transplantation may be necessary.

OTHER SKIN CONDITIONS

LEG BANDS

Q: *Our baby boy has a thin reddish ring around his lower leg. What could have caused this?*

A: What you're describing sounds like *curvilinear lesions,* a harmless condition usually caused by overly snug socks, pants, or sleeves. The tight elastic bands from these or other clothing can cut off circulation and injure a baby's delicate skin. The lesions often start out as red marks around the calves—usually in the exact same place on both legs—and wind up as temporary red bumps. The skin may also turn blue (*cyanotic*) because of the reduced blood supply (see **Blue Skin,** above). When the offending clothing is removed or loosened, the welt will go away.

However, if present at birth, a discolored band can signal a rare, more serious condition, medically known as *amniotic band syndrome* (*ABS*). These bands don't occur only on a newborn's legs or arms; they may show up on any part of the baby's body. And unlike curvilinear lesions, they're not found symmetrically on both sides of the body.

ABS is caused when a part or parts of a baby's body actually gets entangled in the stringlike *amniotic bands* in the womb. This cuts off the blood supply to the developing limbs. Babies with ABS are usually born with other, more obvious signs, such as webbed fingers or toes, deformed nails, and limbs of different lengths.

SWEATY, SALTY SKIN

Q: *When I cuddle and kiss my newborn baby girl, she's often sweaty and her skin tastes salty. Is this normal?*

A: It's not unusual for babies to sweat. Indeed, many parents complain that their babies have sweaty heads. Because their temperature-regulating systems aren't fully developed, babies sweat easily. And because sweat contains a lot of salt, it can taste salty.

Normally, if a baby sweats occasionally, it's nothing to worry about. In fact, the sweat may merely be a warning sign that the baby is overdressed or in an overheated room.

On the other hand, excessive sweating—medically known as *hyperhidrosis*—can signal several potentially serious conditions. These include an overactive thyroid (*hyperthyroidism*), diabetes, asthma, and rickets. However, in all of these disorders, other, more obvious and serious signs than sweating would be noticed.

SPEAKING OF SIGNS

Children in general are over-cloath'd and over-fed . . . to these Causes I impute almost all Diseases . . . they think a new-born Infant cannot be kept too warm; from this Prejudice they load and bind it with Flannels, Wrappers, Swathes, Stays, &c.

—William Cadogan,
British physician, 1748

STOP SIGN

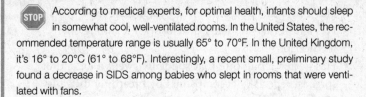

According to medical experts, for optimal health, infants should sleep in somewhat cool, well-ventilated rooms. In the United States, the recommended temperature range is usually 65° to 70°F. In the United Kingdom, it's 16° to 20°C (61° to 68°F). Interestingly, a recent small, preliminary study found a decrease in SIDS among babies who slept in rooms that were ventilated with fans.

If your baby's skin *always* tastes salty, even when she's not sweating, it can be an important early warning sign of *cystic fibrosis* (*CF*), a rare, inherited disease that causes respiratory and gastrointestinal problems in children. Other early signs in infants and babies include breathing difficulties and frequent diarrhea with greasy, foul-smelling stools. (See Chapter 10.) In milder forms of CF, the signs may not show up until the teen years or young adulthood. While there currently is no cure for CF, treatments have improved tremendously in recent years, and life expectancy has increased greatly.

SIGNING OFF

Every baby should have a complete skin exam at birth and have his or her skin carefully examined at every subsequent checkup. But many skin changes and conditions occur between appointments, and parents may be the first ones to spot significant skin signs.

NOTIFY YOUR CHILD'S HEALTHCARE PROVIDER
AS SOON AS POSSIBLE IF YOU NOTICE:

- That your baby's skin has a yellowish tint (jaundice)
- An unusual rash, bruise, discoloration, or lump on or under your baby's skin
- Any change in the color, size, or texture of a birthmark, mole, lump, or bump
- Any birthmark, other mark, mole, lump, or rash on your baby's skin that bleeds, produces pus, looks infected, or itches excessively

NOTIFY YOUR CHILD'S HEALTHCARE PROVIDER
IMMEDIATELY IF YOUR BABY:

- Has a rash that's accompanied by a high fever
- Has a rash that suddenly develops while taking any medication
- Has gotten a bug bite that suddenly swells a lot and/or spreads, especially accompanied by breathing difficulty
- Has prolonged or profuse bleeding from a cut or other wound

A pediatrician can diagnose and treat most skin conditions found in babies. However, some skin disorders may require referral to a pediatric dermatologist, ophthalmologist, neurologist, endocrinologist, or other specialist.

CHAPTER 9

YOUR BABY'S GENITALS

What are little boys made of?
Nails and snails, and puppy-dogs' tails;
That's what little boys are made of.
What are little girls made of?
Sugar and spice, and everything nice;
That's what little girls are made of.
—Popular nursery rhyme

A BABY'S GENDER IS A source of much excited speculation during pregnancy. Expectant parents will often ask their doctor to keep the baby's sex a secret so they can keep on guessing until the newborn makes his or her first appearance. But an infant's sex organs frequently don't look anything like what parents expect. Newborns' genitals may be bruised or swollen for several days from the physical rigors of birth. Or they may be swollen from the remnants of the maternal hormones that circulate to babies in the womb. In most cases, however, a baby's sex organs will look normal in a few days.

Parents of newborns devote much of their attention to their baby's genitals—not only how they look but also what comes out of them. Indeed, a baby's sex organs are no small matter when it comes to health. Their size, shape, and even smell can signal any number of conditions, which can range from insignificant to potentially serious. Parents can even tell how well their baby's urinary system is working by watching him or her urinate, paying attention to the direction in which the pee is pointing, and how much and how fast it flows.

BOY OR GIRL?

Q: My niece gave birth to a baby, but she doesn't know yet if it's a boy or a girl. Her doctor can't even tell her for sure. How could that be, and does it mean the baby might have other problems as well?

A: It sounds like your niece's baby was born with a condition medically known as a *disorder of sexual development (DSD)*. Formerly called *ambiguous genitalia,* DSD is a very rare disorder in which a baby's genitals look different from what would be expected for him or her. For example, a baby girl may be born with an enlarged clitoris that looks like a penis, and/or the lips of her vagina (*labia*) may be fused, resembling a scrotum. A baby boy with DSD may be born with an unusually small penis that looks like a clitoris, and a small scrotum that resembles labia. (See **Little Penis,** below.) And rather than being located at the tip of the penis, the opening to the *urethra* (where the urine comes out) may be found elsewhere on the penis, a condition medically known as *hypospadias*. (See **Peeing Off Center,** below.)

> ### SIGNIFICANT FACT
>
> ⚠ There has been a lot of controversy recently over the various medical terms used to describe genital ambiguity and other genital-related abnormalities, including *ambiguous genitalia*, *intersexuality,* and *pseudo-hermaphroditism*. In 2006 an international panel of experts recommended that the term *disorders of sex development (DSD)* be used instead.

Whether a baby is genetically a boy or girl is determined at conception. However, various hormonal, genetic, chemical, or other factors during pregnancy can disrupt the process that causes fetal tissue to take on the appearance of normal male or female genitalia. Although the specific cause can't always be determined, babies with a family history of this condition are at increased risk, as are babies whose mothers took steroids, progesterone, estrogen, or other hormones during pregnancy.

STOP SIGN

 Whenever there is doubt about a newborn's gender, a pediatric endocrinologist should be consulted immediately.

The leading cause of DSD in girls is *congenital adrenal hyperplasia* (*CAH*), a very rare and potentially very serious genetic disorder. In this condition, the adrenal glands produce too much *androgen* (male sex hormone) but not enough of the hormone *cortisol*. While some male infants with CAH may have an enlarged penis, most will show no early visible signs.

SIGNIFICANT FACT

DSD can cause social and psychological distress for the parents and, later on, the child. It's important, therefore, for the family to work closely with a team of experts, which may include neonatologists, geneticists, ethicists, endocrinologists, surgeons, and psychological counselors.

Most states require newborns to be screened for CAH. Unfortunately, it can go undiagnosed in those states that don't mandate screening, or when babies are born in settings or locales where screening isn't available. Without treatment, which involves replacing the missing hormones, CAH can lead to a life-threatening *adrenal crisis*. Warning signs in infants include weight loss or failure to regain birth weight, lack of appetite, vomiting, and dehydration.

In general, treatment of DSD typically involves hormones and/or reconstructive or other surgery. Counseling is advisable for the family as the child grows older. The good news is that most children with DSD can have normal sex lives, and many will be able to have their own children.

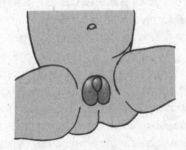

DISORDER OF SEXUAL DEVELOPMENT IN AN INFANT GIRL

VAGINAL VARIATIONS

SWOLLEN VAGINA

Q: *Our baby girl's vagina looks rather large for a baby. Is that normal?*

A: Most, if not all, baby girls are born with swollen *labia* (the lips of the vagina). While in the womb, both baby girls and boys are infused with their mothers' hormones, which results in the swollen breasts and genitals that are so common in newborns. (See Chapter 7.) The vaginal swelling usually resolves in 2 to 4 weeks.

If, however, a baby's vagina remains swollen, it can be a warning sign of a *congenital vaginal obstruction*. This is a rare condition that's usually caused by an *imperforate hymen*. Girls with this condition are born without an opening in their hymen, the thin membrane that covers the entrance to the vagina. This causes fluid to accumulate in the vagina, which in turn causes it to swell. The uterus can sometimes become enlarged as well.

SIGN OF THE TIMES

The word *hymen* comes from the name of the Greek god Hymenaios, god of marriage.

Although it's usually diagnosed soon after birth, an imperforate hymen is sometimes not caught until a girl reaches puberty and fails to menstruate. Treatment in infants typically involves a simple office procedure to open the hymen.

EXTRA PIECE OF SKIN

Q: *I just babysat for my 2-month-old niece. When I changed her diaper, I noticed a piece of skin sticking out of her vagina. What could it be?*

A: It sounds as if your niece has a common condition medically known as a *vaginal tag* or *hymenal tag*. In fact, 1 in 10 girls are born with this extra piece of skin protruding from the vagina. Like enlarged labia (see **Swollen Vagina,** above), these tags are caused by the maternal hormones that reach babies in the womb. They're not only normal, they're also harmless. They usually shrink and recede into the vagina in about 2 to 4 weeks, when the mother's hormones are no longer circulating in the baby's blood. Vaginal tags require no treatment unless they become irritated or bleed from overly vigorous cleaning.

BABY PERIOD

Q: *My new granddaughter just came home from the hospital and I noticed a pinkish discharge in her diaper that looks like blood. My daughter-in-law says that this is perfectly normal in newborn babies. Is she right?*

A: It's very normal for newborn girls to have a vaginal discharge, medically known as *physiologic leukorrhea*. The discharge is caused by the normal drop of the maternal hormones in the baby's bloodstream that occurs after birth. (See **Swollen Vagina,** above.) It can be clear, white, pink, or red. When blood-tinged, it's referred to as *false menstruation*, or more colloquially a *mini-period*. It's similar to menstrual bleeding in adult women, which results from a sudden decrease in estrogen.

Vaginal discharge in a newborn is usually totally benign. It tends to stop in a few days but can sometimes last for up to 2 weeks. If it persists for much longer, it can signal a vaginal infection. (See **Yucky Odor,** below.)

YUCKY ODOR

Q: *Recently, when I change my 2-year-old daughter's diapers, I've noticed an unpleasant odor coming from her vagina. What could be causing this?*

A: A disagreeable vaginal odor is often a sign of a vaginal infection, medically known as *vaginitis* or *vulvovaginitis*. Other signs occasionally include irritation of the skin around the vagina, discharge, and/or itching. (Since your daughter will probably not be able to tell you that she has an itch, watch out for vaginal scratching.) Vaginitis is fairly common in baby girls who aren't toilet-trained and is caused by bacteria from the urine and feces that accumulate in their diapers. Premature and low-birth-weight babies are at increased risk.

Vaginitis can also be a sign that a baby has a skin or other infection.

Because babies like to explore their bodies, especially when their diapers are off, they can easily spread bacteria from their skin, mouths, and noses to their genitals.

Treatment (and prevention) usually involves frequent, careful washing of the baby's bottom with mild soap, along with frequent diaper changes. Bacteria-caused vaginal infections will typically also require treatment with oral or topical antibiotics or other medications.

If the vaginal odor smells like yeast, it may be a sign of *candida,* a fungal (yeast) infection that's quite common in girls younger than 2 years old, as it is in adult women. Also known as *vaginal thrush,* it's caused by the same fungal bacteria that cause oral thrush. (See Chapter 6.) A thick white discharge is another common sign, and itching may also be present (again, look out for excessive scratching). Babies who are treated with antibiotics for other infections are at an increased risk for vaginal thrush, as are those born to mothers who have this infection. While usually of no lasting concern, frequent bouts of candida can be an early warning sign of type 1 (juvenile) diabetes (see Chapter 10) or an underlying problem with the baby's immune system. Candida is commonly treated with antifungal creams.

Last, a very unpleasant vaginal odor in a toddler can be a warning sign that a foreign object is lodged in the vagina. There may also be a brownish discharge, which may signal an infection. All babies love to explore their bodies, and such objects as wads of toilet tissue, beads, small toys, and even crayons often find their way into babies' vaginas, as well as their noses, ears, and mouths. (See Chapters 4 and 5.) Once the offending object is removed by a doctor, the offensive odor will usually quickly disappear. And if there is an infection, it will need to be treated as well.

PENIS PECULIARITIES

PENIS PEARLS

Q: *Our son had a hard white glob on the tip of his penis when he was born. It was gone in a few days. What could it have been?*

A: What you're describing sounds like a *penile pearl*. These tiny, firm, protein-packed bumps at the tip of an uncircumcised penis are akin to *Epstein's pearls,* which are often seen on the gums of newborns and on the roofs of their mouths. (See Chapter 6.) Like Epstein's pearls, penile pearls are common and inconsequential and they will go away on their own in time. They don't even interfere with circumcision or urination.

SNUG FORESKIN

Q: *When I change my son's diaper or bathe him, I find it difficult to push back his foreskin to clean him. What could be causing this?*

A: It's very common and normal for newborns to have a tight foreskin—medically called *phimosis*. In fact, only about 4% of newborns have a foreskin that can be fully pushed back. But as a boy grows, so will his penis; by age 3, most boys have a foreskin that can be moved back and forth completely and easily.

Phimosis can also be acquired after birth, in which case it may be a

---

WARNING SIGN

 Excessive force should never be used to push back a foreskin. This can lead to *paraphimosis,* a medical emergency in which the foreskin gets stuck, constricting and damaging the delicate penis.

sign of poor hygiene. *Smegma*—a milky, sticky substance made up of dead skin cells and natural secretions—can accumulate under the foreskin. As it dries it becomes firm and cheeselike and can restrict the movement of the foreskin. Another possible cause of phimosis is a chronic infection of the penis called *balanoposthitis*. (See **Smelly Penis,** below.) In this case, treatment with antibiotics or other medications and careful attention to hygiene are usually recommended.

Sometimes a tight foreskin can cause pain or trouble urinating, both of which can signal an obstruction. In these cases, circumcision may be recommended.

SMELLY PENIS

Q: *I've noticed that my 14-month-old son's penis has a peculiar odor. Could it be an infection?*

A: In uncircumcised boys, an offensive genital odor may be a sign of *posthitis,* an inflammation of the foreskin. And in both circumcised and uncircumcised boys it can be a sign of *balanitis,* an inflammation of the *glans* (the head of the penis) that is commonly seen in babies with diaper rash. Balanitis requires immediate attention and is usually treated with antibiotics. When both the foreskin and the glans are inflamed, it's appropriately called *balanoposthitis.*

Other signs of penile inflammation, which is often caused by poor hygiene, are redness, swelling, and pain. It can also lead to itching, so you may notice that your son scratches his genital area. All of these signs can point to a yeast or bacterial infection. If there is an infection, antifungal or antibiotic medication may be recommended.

STOP SIGN

STOP   Keeping a baby's bottom and hands very clean is the best way to prevent genital and urinary tract infections. Toilet-trained toddlers should wear only 100% cotton underpants.

CROOKED PENIS

Q: *Our baby's penis looks bent. Can this create problems for him?*

A: A curved or bent penis is medically called *chordee* (aka *dorsal hood deformity*). It's most often seen in boys with *hypospadias,* a relatively common condition in which the opening of the penis is misplaced. (See **Peeing Off Center,** below.) Chordee is usually the result of a less-than-normal amount of skin on the penis.

Chordee isn't always obvious. Indeed, some parents may not notice it until their baby boy has an erection that's not straight. (See **Penis Play,** below.) In some cases, surgery is required to correct the curvature. If untreated, severe chordee impairs the ability to engage in sexual intercourse in adulthood.

> **SIGN OF THE TIMES**
>
> The incidence of congenital anomalies of the penis has been on the rise over the last few decades. Hypospadias, chordee, or a combination of the 2 now make up more than 80% of these penile problems. Some researchers believe pollutants may be to blame.

LITTLE PENIS

Q: *Our newborn grandson's penis seems very small. Our daughter says he's perfectly normal. Should I be concerned?*

A: In a newborn, a normal-sized penis is really quite small, measuring just over 1 inch to 1¾ inches from tip to base. Only when it's under

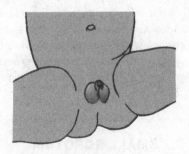

MICROPENIS

about ¾ of an inch at birth is a penis considered medically to be small and referred to as a *micropenis* or *microphallus*. In most boys, these tiny penises are normally formed, just abnormally short. That said, some babies with very small penises will also have *hypospadias*. (See **Peeing Off Center,** below.)

Sometimes what appears to be a small penis is actually a *hidden penis,* a condition in which a pudgy baby boy's belly fat covers up his normal-sized penis. In these cases, the "innie" penis may poke out only when the baby urinates or gets an erection (see **Penis Play,** below). A hidden penis may resolve on its own as the baby loses weight or gets older. If not, surgery may be recommended. In rare cases, a penis that's not prominent can also be a sign of a *congenital buried penis,* a condition in which an otherwise normal penis is partially or completely concealed in the baby's abdominal tissues at birth. Surgery is recommended to correct this type of problem.

> ### SIGNIFICANT FACT
>
> ⚠ The penis grows less than ½ inch (1 cm) during the first 3 to 4 years after birth.

A true micropenis can be a sign of hormonal or other disorders, including *Klinefelter syndrome.* (See Chapter 9 and **Small Scrotum,** below.) In very rare cases, a penis can be so small that the baby's sex isn't obvious. The penis may even resemble a clitoris. A baby with a micropenis should undergo chromosomal and/or endocrine testing to help clarify any uncertainty about gender and sexual development.

> ### WARNING SIGN
>
> 🔔 An enlarged penis and/or testicle can be signs of *precocious puberty,* the early development of puberty, usually before 9 years of age. All boys with an enlarged penis or testicles should be evaluated to distinguish between true precocious puberty, which can signal a hormonal or other disorder requiring immediate treatment, and partial precocious puberty, which is usually a condition that doesn't require treatment.

SMALL SCROTUM

Q: Our newborn son's scrotum seems unusually small. Our other son's scrotum didn't seem like that at birth. Could something be wrong?

A: Your son may have what's medically known as an *undescended testicle* or *cryptorchidism,* a condition that's fairly common in newborns. During fetal development, the testicles—the organs responsible for making male hormones and sperm—are in the abdomen. Just before or soon after birth, they move down into the scrotum. When a testicle fails to descend, it's fittingly referred to as undescended. While only one testis is usually affected (most often the left), occasionally both testes fail to descend.

About 4% of newborns will have at least one undescended testicle, making it the most common congenital genital abnormality in boys. Premature and low-birth-weight baby boys are at increased risk for undescended testicles, as are boys with certain rare types of congenital and genetic syndromes.

Fortunately, in about 75% of babies with this condition, the testicle moves down into the scrotum within the first few months of life. If that doesn't happen, treatment with hormones and/or a simple surgical procedure is needed within the first year of life.

Undescended testicles can be an early warning sign of Klinefelter syndrome, a chromosomal disorder that can cause delayed puberty and fertil-

> ### SIGNIFICANT FACT
>
> It's important that undescended testicles be fixed. At 12 months of age, a boy with an undescended testicle can start to lose his ability to make sperm. And as an adult he would be at increased risk of testicular cancer. Correcting the problem before puberty lowers that risk.

ity problems in later life. Other signs may include a small penis and hypospadias. (See Chapter 7 and **Little Penis,** above.)

As odd as it may seem, some boys have testicles that occasionally and temporarily recede back into the abdomen. Medically known as *retractile testes,* this is a normal phenomenon. Unlike undescended testes, which can have serious consequences if they don't correct themselves or receive treatment, sporadic retractile testes don't require medical attention.

BULGING SCROTUM

Q: *My sister told me that my 9-month-old nephew has an inguinal hernia. My son had an umbilical hernia. Are they the same?*

A: In boys, an *inguinal hernia* is a soft and generally painless bulge in the scrotum or groin. While an umbilical hernia happens when part of the abdomen or its lining bulges through the area around the belly button (see Chapter 7), an inguinal hernia arises when some tissue—usually part of the *peritoneum* (the membrane that covers the abdominal cavity)—pokes through the pathway that the testicles used in their descent into the scrotum. (In girls, an inguinal hernia can appear anywhere from the groin to the vagina.) Like umbilical hernias, inguinal ones can get bigger and more noticeable when a baby cries or coughs. Indeed, many parents first notice an inguinal hernia when their baby is standing up, or when he strains while having a bowel movement.

Inguinal hernias are fairly common in babies—as many as 5% of baby boys have them—and they tend to run in families. Premature and low-birth-weight babies, particularly boys, are at increased risk. Most of these hernias show up on the right side, but in about 10% of cases the baby will have a hernia on both sides of the groin (*bilateral hernia*) at the same time. This is more prevalent in preemies.

DANGER SIGN

An inguinal hernia that suddenly enlarges and causes vomiting and obvious pain can signal that part of the intestine has become trapped in the abdominal wall (an *incarcerated hernia*). If left untreated, this condition can lead to an even more serious situation—a *strangulated hernia*. In these cases, blood supply to the intestinal tissue is cut off. This is a medical emergency requiring surgery. Incarcerated hernias are more common in girls, in premature babies, and in the first 6 months of life.

Baby boys with inguinal hernias often have other genital-related disorders, including *undescended testicles* (see **Small Scrotum,** above) and *hypospadias,* another fairly common condition in which the opening of the penis is misplaced, usually on the underside rather than on

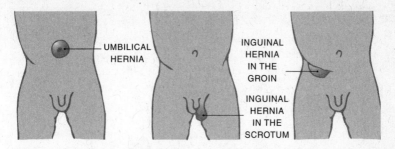

DIFFERENT TYPES OF HERNIAS

the tip. (See **Peeing Off Center,** below.) Children with *congenital hip dislocation* (see Chapter 7) and *cystic fibrosis* (see Chapter 8) are also at increased risk for inguinal hernias.

In many cases of inguinal hernia, the protrusion can actually be pushed back into place. Whether or not they can be pushed back, inguinal hernias in babies are easily treated surgically.

SIGN OF THE TIMES

In the 17th century, a popular hernia treatment was to give a child a tonic made from various herbs. One key ingredient was rupturewort (*Herniaria glabra*), a plant still used today as a diuretic and antispasmodic.

SWOLLEN SCROTUM

Q: While babysitting for our 6-month-old grandson, my husband and I noticed that his scrotum was very large. It doesn't seem to bother him—or our daughter, who says it's nothing to worry about. What could be causing this swelling? Should we be worried?

A: A swollen scrotum may be a sign of a *hydrocele,* which forms when the fluid-filled sac that surrounds the testes during their normal descent from the abdomen into the scrotum doesn't drain properly or when fluid builds up in the scrotum. Many boys—although how many is unclear—are born with hydroceles. In some babies, this condition may not be noticed for several months.

In general, hydroceles, which can affect one or both testicles, are benign and painless. Many doctors describe the scrotum of a baby with a hydrocele as having the feel of a "water balloon." Other signs may include a scrotum that fluctuates in size or one that has a bluish tint.

Most hydroceles disappear on their own before the baby's first birthday. But if a hydrocele causes discomfort or disfigurement, or is so large that it's in danger of impairing the blood supply to the testicle, it may need to be surgically repaired.

PEEING OFF CENTER

Q: We've noticed that when our infant son pees, it seems like the urine doesn't spout from the tip of his penis. Can this be a problem?

A: What you're describing sounds like a condition called *hypospadias,* in which the opening of the *urethra* (the tubelike structure inside the penis that carries urine out from the bladder) is on the underside of the shaft of the penis rather than in its normal position at the tip (*glans*). Indeed, sometimes the opening is so far back that it's behind the scrotum. (There is another, far less common type of congenital misplacement of the urethra in boys, medically known as *epispadias,* in which the opening is on the top side of the penis.)

Hypospadias is one of the most common birth defects, occurring in 8 out of every 1,000 boys. Although usually noticed at birth, the abnormality is sometimes so subtle that it's not detected until later. Hypospadias tends to run in families. A baby whose brother or father had hypospadias is at an increased risk of being born with it too.

Hypospadias can point to a number of other genital-related conditions. About 10% of boys who have it will also have an *inguinal hernia,* and a smaller number will also have a *hydrocele.* (See **Bulging Scrotum** and **Swollen Scrotum,** above.) Babies born with hypospadias may also have penises that curve downward. Medically referred to as *chordee,* this

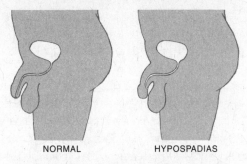

NORMAL   HYPOSPADIAS

NORMAL AND ABNORMAL URETHRAL OPENING

is particularly common when the urethral opening is located far down the penis, away from the glans. (See **Crooked Penis,** above.)

WARNING SIGN

Designer toilet seats can be dangerous for toilet-trained toddlers. There have been several reports about heavy wooden or other ornamental toilet seats falling down on boys' penises.

Hypospadias can be repaired surgically. Without surgery, babies may experience what doctors call a *urine stream deformity,* which makes it difficult for them to pee in a straight line. As a result, a boy with this condition may have to urinate while sitting rather than standing, which can be very embarrassing as he grows older. (See **Missing the Mark,** below.)

Depending on where the urethral opening is on the penis, surgery may be recommended. If the problem is noticed at birth, circumcision should be delayed; the foreskin may be needed to help repair the urethra, particularly if the penis is also curved.

MISSING THE MARK

Q: Our son's potty-trained, but when he urinates, pee often winds up around, rather than in, the potty. What could be the problem?

A: In toilet-trained boys, a urine stream that goes askew may be a subtle sign of hypospadias. (See **Peeing Off Cen-**

SIGN OF THE TIMES

Potties have been used for toilet-training toddlers as far back as the 5th century B.C., if not before. Ancient Greek pottery has been unearthed that depicts babies sitting on potties, dangling their legs, and waving little rattles.

ter, above.) But if the urinary stream seems more like a fine spray than a spurt, it may signal *meatal stenosis,* a very small urethral opening. Another telltale sign of this condition is if a boy takes longer to empty his bladder than others his age.

Meatal stenosis is usually an acquired problem in boys. It occurs when the urethral opening becomes inflamed or scarred—most likely after genital surgery or injury, or after a baby's had a urinary catheter in place for some time. It's far more common in boys who've been circumcised than in those who have not—the delicate tip of a circumcised penis can easily become irritated, particularly from a urine-drenched diaper. To help prevent difficulty urinating, an office procedure to increase the size of the urethral opening may be required.

GENITAL-RELATED BEHAVIOR

GENITAL TOUCHING

Q: Our 22-month-old daughter loves to take off her diaper and run around naked. She also occasionally touches her vagina. Is this normal?

A: It's perfectly normal for baby girls and boys not only to enjoy running around naked but to touch their genitals as well. Babies learn about their world by using all their senses, and touching is one of their very favorites. Babies use their fingers to explore every nook, cranny, and protruding body part. This includes vaginas in girls and penises in boys.

Many parents worry that this behavior is the same thing as masturbation. But while babies usually find it pleasurable to touch their genitals, this touching doesn't have the same sexual meaning that it does for older children and adults.

PENIS PLAY

Q: We're adopting our first baby—a newborn boy. We've read that baby boys get erections. Is that true?

A: Yes, it's perfectly normal for new-born boys—and older boys, for that matter—to get erections. In fact, this is a healthy sign that the nerves to the penis are functioning properly.

In infants, erections are not sexually driven. For example, a full bladder is a common cause of erections in babies (as well as in adults). Erections might also arise from normal stimulation that can occur when a baby boy's penis rubs against his diapers or underpants. And babies usually leave no appendage unexplored—their penises are no exception. Penis touching and play is a very normal, harmless, and universal practice (see **Genital Touching,** above). Baby erections usually last a couple of minutes and disappear when any stimulating trigger is removed. On the other hand, parents should not be alarmed if they do not notice erections. Erections often occur without being spotted by the mother or father.

DANGER SIGN

 An erection lasting several hours in babies and toddlers—a condition called *priapism*—is a medical emergency. Without immediate treatment, the delicate structure of the penis can be permanently damaged, leading to erectile dysfunction later in life.

DIAPER DUMPING

Q: *I'm a nanny for a toddler who likes to hide things down his diaper. I'm afraid he's going to hurt himself. Am I being overly cautious?*

DANGER SIGN

 Any boy whose foreskin gets stuck when pushed back (*paraphimosis*) should be checked to be certain that no foreign objects—such as strands of hair, pieces of clothing, or rubber bands—are trapped under the foreskin or around the penis. If the object remains, it can lead to infection. Worse, it can cut off blood supply to the penis, which is a medical emergency.

A: It's not unusual for children to use their diapers as their personal tote bags, so it's important to be certain that no potentially harmful item—pins, beads, even food—makes its way down the diaper chute. Strands of string and long hair can be particularly dangerous. If they get wrapped around a baby boy's penis, they can cause what doctors call *hair-thread tourniquet syndrome,* cutting off the blood supply to the delicate organ. This can cause permanent damage.

SIGNING OFF

At the time of delivery, a baby's genitals will be carefully evaluated for anatomical or other abnormalities. If there is any abnormality or doubt about a baby's gender, a pediatric endocrinologist should be consulted immediately. But some genital-related problems may not show up until the baby is at home. And even though a baby's genitals will be examined again at each well-baby visit to the pediatrician, various conditions can crop up at any time. Some may be benign, but some may require prompt medical attention.

NOTIFY YOUR CHILD'S HEALTHCARE PROVIDER AS SOON AS POSSIBLE IF YOU NOTICE YOUR BABY'S GENITALS:

- Have suddenly become swollen
- Have a puslike, bloody, or foul-smelling discharge
- Have bruises or cuts

NOTIFY YOUR CHILD'S HEALTHCARE PROVIDER IMMEDIATELY OR GO TO THE EMERGENCY ROOM IF YOUR BABY:

- Is bleeding a lot from the penis or vagina
- Has a hernia or lump in the groin and suddenly starts vomiting and/or appears to be in pain
- Is crying uncontrollably while clutching his or her genitals

A pediatrician can diagnose and treat most genital-related conditions found in babies. However, some disorders may require referral to a pediatric specialist in neonatology, endocrinology, gynecology, urology, or cosmetic surgery. For certain medical problems, the family may be referred to a geneticist, ethicist, and/or therapist.

CHAPTER 10

········

YOUR BABY'S BODY WASTES

A baby is an alimentary canal
with a loud voice at one end and
no responsibility at the other.
—Ronald Reagan, actor
and U.S. president

THROUGHOUT THE AGES, THE COLOR, fragrance, and frequency of a baby's urine and feces have fascinated parents, physicians, and even soothsayers. To this day, a peek at poop and pee can give parents and pediatricians a plentitude of information about the baby's health.

YOUR BABY'S URINE

Urine goes by a wide variety of names, both naughty and nice. Regardless of what they call it, parents should periodically take a peek inside their baby's wet diapers or—if their child is toilet-trained—the potty. They can learn a great deal by keeping an eye on and occasionally sniffing their baby's urine.

SIGN OF THE TIMES

In medieval times, medical practitioners called "pisse prophets" not only examined urine for signs of illness but perused it to predict the future. And because urine often had a golden yellow color, alchemists believed that gold could be extracted from it.

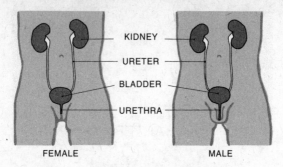

URINARY TRACT ANATOMY

The urinary tract includes several organs and functions. Here they are:

- *Kidneys*—collect wastes and extra water from the blood to make urine
- *Ureters*—carry urine from the kidneys to the bladder
- *Bladder*—stores urine and squeezes it out when full
- *Urethra*—carries urine out of the bladder when urinating

A WEE BIT OF PEE

Q: *In babysitting class we learned that it's normal to change a baby's wet diaper at least 6 to 8 times a day. I take care of a 6-month-old baby girl, and recently I've needed to change her only a few times a day. Could there be a problem?*

A: Unless you're with a baby 24 hours a day, it's difficult to know exactly how many times a day he or she actually urinates. Although most babies urinate between 6 and 12 times a day, there are individual differences. For example, babies who drink a lot will pee a lot, while those who drink relatively little will pee less. And babies (and adults) tend to pee less in hot weather because the excess fluid is sweated out.

HEALTHY SIGNS

Urine in a healthy baby (and adult) is clear or slightly yellow, odorless, and not foamy or frothy. It's also sterile.

That said, a decrease in urine output, medically known as *oliguria,* can be a warning sign of *dehydration,* the loss of body fluids. Several situations and sicknesses can cause a child to become dehydrated, including being extremely overheated, having a high fever, vomiting, and diarrhea (see **Watery Stools,** below). Acting very thirsty and having dark yellow or smelly urine are early signs of dehydration. (See **Very Yellow Pee** and **Not-So-Sweet Pee,** below.) Other common signs include sunken "soft spots" (see Chapter 1), sunken eyes, diminished tears, dry lips and mouth, and a furry tongue. The baby's skin may also look mottled or grayish and be cool to the touch. Fortunately, dehydration can be averted—and even reversed—if fluids are replenished at the first signs of danger.

Two important causes of dehydration in children are diarrhea and vomiting. A common cause of diarrhea (see **Watery Stools,** below)—and subsequently dehydration—is *gastroenteritis,* a usually self-limiting infection of the gastrointestinal tract that is typically caused by a virus. Vomiting can accompany almost any gastrointestinal illness and may also occur with a urinary tract infection.

Infrequent urination can also be a sign of some serious kidney problems or an obstruction somewhere along the urinary tract. Other signs of an obstruction are a urine stream that isn't very strong or pee that just dribbles out.

A urinary obstruction can occur for several reasons, including a misplaced or narrow ureter or urethra or a kidney stone. Depending on where the obstruction is located along the urinary tract, treatment may range from medication to a simple office procedure or more extensive surgery. If left untreated, a urinary obstruction can lead to permanent kidney damage or failure.

PEEING A LOT

Q: *Our 1-year-old son seems to pee all the time lately. What could be causing this?*

A: Urinating more than usual may be a sign that a baby is drinking a lot of liquids that have a diuretic effect, especially tea, cranberry juice, and cola drinks. Or it may be a tip-off that a child is eating a lot of salty foods, which are causing him or her to drink more liquids than usual.

Frequent urination is also an important warning sign of a *urinary tract infection* (*UTI*). Other signs include urine that has an off smell (see **Not-So-Sweet Pee,** below) and cloudy, dark yellow, or reddish urine (see **Very Yellow Pee** and **Reddish or Pinkish Pee Spots,** below).

An increase in urinary frequency that occurs with an increase in thirst may also be a red flag for *type 1 diabetes mellitus* (*DM 1*), which used to be called *juvenile diabetes* and is sometimes referred to as *sugar diabetes.* In this condition, which is rare in babies, the body doesn't produce enough insulin and/or use it properly. This results in abnormally high levels of *glucose* (sugar) in the bloodstream. Other common signs of DM 1 in babies include constant hunger, weight loss, fatigue, and vomiting. The baby may also have sweet-smelling urine, especially in more serious or uncontrolled cases.

DM 1 is an autoimmune disorder that affects about 1 in 600 children, usually between the ages of 6 and 12. Children with other autoimmune diseases, such as *hyperthyroidism* (see

SIGNIFICANT FACTS

Type 1 diabetes is an autoimmune disorder that tends to affect children and young adults. It's a totally different disorder from type 2 diabetes, the most common form. Type 2, which used to be seen mostly in adults and was referred to as adult-onset diabetes, has increased dramatically in children. While sugar levels are too high in both types, only type 2 is related to diet and obesity.

Chapter 3) and *celiac disease* (see **Watery Stools** and **Recurrent Runs,** below), are at increased risk. Sometimes DM 1 also runs in families. Unfortunately, the incidence of type 1 diabetes in children is on the rise. And it's increasing fastest among preschool children—at an alarming rate of 5% a year. This increase is believed to be the result of environmental factors.

Without treatment, which involves daily shots of insulin, DM 1 can cause damage to many vital parts of the body, including the heart, kidneys, eyes, blood vessels, and nerves. And babies with this disease can develop *diabetic ketoacidosis* (*DKA*), a potentially life-threatening condition.

WARNING SIGN

Any baby who has been urinating a lot and has been excessively thirsty for several days should have his or her urine tested for glucose as soon as possible by a doctor. If there is no glucose in the urine, the baby may have diabetes insipidus, which can be life threatening if not treated immediately.

A baby who suddenly has a lot of unusually wet diapers and is extremely thirsty may have a much rarer form of diabetes, *diabetes insipidus* (*DI*), commonly called water diabetes. Totally unrelated to diabetes mellitus, DI is caused by an inadequate production of *antidiuretic hormone* (*ADH*), the hormone that helps balance the amount of water in urine and blood. As a result, the baby's urine becomes very diluted, containing mostly water.

WARNING SIGN

Children who suddenly become diabetic may vomit continuously and be misdiagnosed as having a gastrointestinal infection or the flu. However, a baby with one of these conditions would urinate *less* than usual (because of dehydration), while a baby with diabetes urinates *more* than usual. Without prompt treatment with insulin, the baby may develop DKA and lapse into *diabetic coma,* which is life threatening.

Vigorous nursing with vomiting is another early warning sign of DI in babies. Other signs may include fever, irritability, and constipation from dehydration (see **Periodic Pooping,** below).

If a baby is born with DI, he or she has probably inherited it. Known by

SIGN OF THE TIMES

Diabetes insipidus is believed to have originated in Scotland. According to Scottish folklore, a traveling Gypsy asked a housewife for water for her thirsty son. When the woman refused, the Gypsy cast a spell on her: Her sons would always be thirsty and her daughters would pass the curse on to all future generations.

the politically incorrect term *Gypsy's curse DI,* inherited DI affects more boys than girls.

DI can also be acquired at any age, sometimes as a result of damage to the kidneys or the pituitary gland. Acquired DI can also be caused by a central nervous system tumor. About 25% of the time, though, the cause remains unknown.

Although there's no cure for DI, effective treatments, which include medication and special diets, are available. With treatment, most children can live virtually normal lives. Without it, a baby with the disease may become dangerously dehydrated and fail to thrive.

SPEAKING OF SIGNS

- The word *diabetes,* which was first used in 1425, is derived from the Greek word *diabainein,* which means "standing with legs apart" (as in peeing) and "go through" (as in flowing).
- The *mellitus* in *diabetes mellitus* is Latin for "honey," and the *insipidus* in *diabetes insipidus* is Latin for "without taste." Indeed, the urine of people with diabetes mellitus contains glucose and can actually taste and smell like sugar, while the urine of a person with diabetes insipidus contains mostly water and is, therefore, odorless.

VERY YELLOW PEE

Q: *We've recently noticed that the urine of our 2-year-old daughter is much more yellow-colored than usual. Could this be caused by jaundice or some other problem?*

A: Yellow urine, like orange (see **Orange Pee,** below) and other oddly colored urine, can be a benign sign that a baby is drinking or eating large quantities of foods or beverages of that color. In these cases, the colored pee is temporary—when the baby's diet returns to normal, the urine will also return to its normal, nearly colorless state. Very yellow urine can also be an early warning sign of dehydration, which can be caused by not drinking enough fluids or by excessive sweating from being overheated.

However, urine that looks very yellow can, indeed, be a warning sign of jaundice. A baby with jaundice is also likely to have yellow eyes and skin (see Chapters 3 and 8) and pale stools (see **Pale Poop,** below). While jaundice in newborns is normal, jaundice in older babies can be a sign of liver disease, ranging from mild to serious.

ORANGE PEE

Q: *Our 8-month-old has started to pee orange. She's drinking plenty of liquids, so I know she's not dehydrated. What could it be?*

A: If your baby is drinking a lot of carrot juice, it might explain why her urine is a bit orange. The same goes if she is eating or drinking other foods and beverages that contain beta-carotene, such as pumpkins and squash. These orange-colored foods can also cause a baby's stools and skin to take on a tangerine tinge. (See Chapter 8 and **Orange Poop,** below.)

Another totally benign cause of a slightly orange urine stain in a diaper is a reaction between the normal substances in the baby's urine and the chemicals in the fibers of the diaper. (See **Reddish or Pinkish Pee Spots,** below.) Certain antibiotics, such as rifampin, can also turn pee (and poop) orange. (See **Orange Poop,** below.)

Fortunately, most urine color changes in babies are harmless and are caused by the ingestion of certain foods or drugs. Once a baby cuts down on the colorful culprits in his or her diet, the urine will quickly return to being colorless or light yellow.

REDDISH OR PINKISH PEE SPOTS

Q: *I noticed dark pink urine stains on my 2-month-old son's diaper. I'm concerned that it might be blood. Could it be?*

A: Seeing spots like this in a dirty or clean diaper can certainly be alarming. But if the stains in your son's diaper were blood, they would probably be a brighter red. In a recently circumcised baby, for example, a small amount of fresh, bright red urine would likely signal (normal) bleeding. (The amount of blood following a circumcision typically lessens and disappears in a couple of days.)

SIGN OF THE TIMES

A mid-19th-century medical textbook claimed that black urine in a child with fever preceded epilepsy and that eating rhubarb would prevent it.

Wine-hued urine can also be a telltale sign that the child has been drinking beverages or eating foods that have red dye in them. Cherry-flavored juices, beverages, and gelatin are prime culprits, but eating naturally red foods, such as berries and rhubarb, can also be to blame. Another food-related cause of red-tinted urine is the aptly named and inconsequential condition called *beeturia*. Not surprisingly, this is seen in babies (and adults) after eating beets.

In newborns, reddish or rust-colored residue in a wet disposable diaper may be the result of left-behind uric acid crystals. Newborns have high levels of uric acid in their urine, and when the superabsorbent chemicals in disposable diapers mix with it, they wick away the liquid, leaving behind pink crystals or fine powder. Called *brick dust,* this residue is fairly common in newborn breast-fed babies before their mothers' milk comes in. As babies get older and the level of uric acid in their urine drops, there will be less brick dust. On the other hand, there may be more if a child becomes dehydrated. In rare cases, brick dust can be a sign of a condition called *red-diaper syndrome,* which is usually caused by a gastrointestinal infection with *Serratia marcescens,* a red-pigmented bacterium.

SWEET PEE

Q: *I just gave birth and someone in my new-mothers' group said that there's a serious disease in newborns that causes a baby's urine to smell sweet, like maple syrup. Is this true?*

A: Indeed, there is a very rare, life-threatening, hereditary condition called *maple syrup urine disease* (*MSUD*), which causes a baby's urine to smell exceedingly sweet. Newborns are often screened for it.

Babies with MSUD are missing important protein-processing enzymes. There are different forms of this disease. In the classic, most serious form, children become progressively sick within the first few days of life and may even die. In the less serious and intermittent forms, children are well most of the time but have bouts of sweet-smelling urine and vomiting at certain times, such as when they're sick. This milder type of MSUD most likely will not be picked up by newborn screening. In both the classic and intermittent forms of MSUD, treatment—which includes a lifelong special diet as well as medications—can help prevent or diminish developmental delays or other neurological and medical problems that can develop.

MSUD is an exceedingly rare genetic disorder, occurring in approximately 1 in 100,000 to 185,000 births. However, it's much more common in children of Amish and Mennonite descent. Their rates can be as high as 1 in 380 births.

SIGNIFICANT FACT

While all states require that newborns be tested for metabolic disorders, less than half screen for *maple syrup urine disease* (*MSUD*). If you're not sure that your newborn was screened for MSUD, ask the pediatrician. He or she can arrange screening.

SIGN OF THE TIMES

As far back as 600 B.C., physicians would taste a patient's urine as a part of the diagnostic process. If it was sweet, they knew something was wrong. Sweet-tasting (and -smelling) urine is now a recognized sign of diabetes.

NOT-SO-SWEET PEE

Q: *I've recently noticed that our toddler's urine has an odd, unpleasant smell. What could be causing this?*

Before the discovery of antibiotics, a variety of remedies were used to treat urinary tract infections.

- In ancient Egypt, papyrus cooked in oil was placed on the baby's belly. If that didn't work, the baby was forced to eat a cooked mouse.
- The ancient Greeks favored herbs and bed rest.
- In the 19th century, the treatments of choice included herbal enemas and douches, bleeding, cupping, and even leeches. Indeed, a common treatment for UTIs in young girls consisted of placing the leeches on the unfortunate girl's vulva.

A: Although urine is generally odorless, it will develop a stinky smell—like ammonia—if it sits around for too long in a diaper or potty. Unpleasant-smelling urine can also be a sign of dehydration, in which case the urine might be dark yellow in color. (See **Very Yellow Pee,** above.) And certain foods, such as asparagus, can also give urine an off odor.

But smelly urine, especially if it's cloudy, can be a telltale sign of a *urinary tract infection* (*UTI*). Frequent peeing may also be a sign of a UTI, which is one of the most common infections in babies. (See **Peeing a Lot** and **Very Yellow Pee,** above.)

There are many other signs that typically accompany a UTI, but not all children who have a UTI will show all or even most of them. Toddlers with a UTI may keep acting as though they need to pee or may seem to hesitate a bit before actually peeing. They may clutch their stomachs and grimace or cry while urinating. And they may appear to have pain in the abdomen, side, or back. In younger babies, UTI signs can include loss of appetite, vomiting, irritability, and fever—signs so subtle that they are sometimes ignored or misinterpreted.

WARNING SIGN

Frequent UTIs can be a sign *and* a cause of *urinary reflux* (aka *vesicoureteral reflux*), the backup of urine from the bladder into the ureters during urination. In fact, about half of infants with a UTI have some amount of urine reflux. It affects more newborn boys than girls, but it's more common in girls after the newborn period.

Urinary tract infections are very common in babies and young children, but some are at greater risk than others. For example, uncircumcised boys, particularly those younger than 3 months, are at increased risk because of the way urine flows beneath the foreskin. But in babies older than 3 months, UTIs are more common in girls than in boys. The reason: Their urethras are very short, giving bacteria from the bowel easy access to the bladder. UTIs, which may recur, are usually treated with oral antibiotics.

> **WARNING SIGN**
>
> Canadian researchers have recently found that excessive crying for no apparent reason in infants is likely to be serious in only 1 in 20 cases. But the most common serious problem was urinary tract infection.

THE SCOOP ON BABY POOP

While visitors are busy oohing and aahing at a baby's adorable face, the parents may have their attention focused on something quite different—the infant's feces. From the all-important first bowel movement (*meconium*) to mustard-colored stool, runaway diarrhea, tiny pebblelike poop, and a multitude of other varieties, a baby's feces are bound to fascinate his or her parents . . . and for good reason. The shape, smell, color, consistency, frequency, and quantity of a baby's bowel movements can all reveal a heap of information about his or her health. Studying your baby's stool and other body wastes is definitely *not* a waste of time.

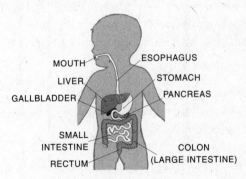

MOUTH
ESOPHAGUS
LIVER
STOMACH
GALLBLADDER
PANCREAS
SMALL
INTESTINE
RECTUM
COLON
(LARGE INTESTINE)

DIGESTIVE TRACT ANATOMY

COLOR CHANGES

YELLOWISH POOP

Q: *Our newborn's bowel movements are quite yellow. Might this be caused by jaundice?*

A: Neonatal jaundice is very common in newborns and is usually harmless. While yellowish eyes, skin, and urine are typical signs of neonatal and other kinds of jaundice (see Chapters 3 and 8), yellow stools are not. Rather, it's pale, chalk-colored stools that are a major warning sign of jaundice and other liver disease. (See **Pale Poop,** below.)

For a couple of days after a baby expels all the meconium—the greenish-black, icky, sticky stuff that's a newborn's first bowel movement—he or she will likely have soft yellowish or greenish stools. The color (and texture) of the baby's bowel movements will then change, depending on his or her diet. The stools of breast-fed babies will be yellowish or a light mustard color with a seedy texture, while those of bottle-fed babies will usually be a darker mustard color with a firmer texture. By the time babies turn 6 months old, most will have more normal-looking brown stools.

ORANGE POOP

Q: *Our 8-month-old daughter has been having orange-colored stools. What could be causing this?*

A: Orange and other oddly colored stools are often the result of diet and are usually totally benign. As the saying goes, "What goes in one end comes out the other." Some of the first solids that are typically given to babies are orange-colored: carrots, sweet potatoes, apricots, mangoes, and pumpkin. Rich in beta-carotene (vitamin A), an important antioxidant found in orange food, these foods will temporarily turn stools orange. A baby's skin and urine may have an orangish hue for the same reason. (See Chapter 8 and **Orange Pee,** above.) Foods containing orange dye, such as orange gelatin or punch, can have the same effect. Orange stools can also result from an excess of beta-carotene or vitamin A in supplements. And babies who have been given the antibiotic *rifampin,* which is used to treat certain bacterial infections, may have orange poop *and* pee. (See **Orange Pee,** above.)

GREEN POOP

Q: I heard that if a baby has green poop, it's a sign of an infection. Is that true?

A: Green stools, like orange ones (see **Orange Poop,** above), may be a perfectly benign sign. Breast-fed ba-

> **HEALTHY SIGN**
>
> Once babies are weaned from the breast or bottle and are eating a normal diet, their stools should have the consistency of a ripe banana, the shape of a sausage, and the color of a cooked hamburger.

bies often have greenish stools, as do babies who eat an abundance of green vegetables, which are naturally rich in chlorophyll (the green pigment found in plants). Lime-flavored gelatin and beverages can also turn a baby's stools green. And green stools can be a telltale sign that a baby has been given iron supplements, certain antibiotics, or laxatives.

When the stools come out quickly (as in diarrhea), they will often be green. Indeed, green stools can be a warning sign of a gastrointestinal infection. Once the infection is treated (either on its own or through medication), the green color will likely clear up too.

PALE POOP

Q: Lately, our 2-month-old daughter's bowel movements have been almost white. Could something be wrong with her?

A: As with other strangely colored stools (see **Orange Poop** and **Green Poop,** above), pale stools can be diet-related. They may mean, for example, that a baby has been eating a lot of white or light-colored food, such as rice, potatoes, or tapioca. Certain penicillins, some anti-diarrhea medicines such as Kaopectate, and other drugs can have the same effect.

However, persistently pale poop may be a telltale sign of some serious disorders. Stools get their brown color from *bile,* a greenish fluid produced by the liver that helps digest fats and excrete toxins. When the bile is not adequately produced or is blocked from reaching the intestines, the stools turn pale, claylike, or chalklike in color. This is medically known as *acholic stools*. Acholic stools can be a warning sign of liver disorders, especially in babies who have jaundice (yellow eyes and skin and dark yellow urine) that persists longer than the normal and benign neonatal jaundice. (See Chapters 3 and 8.)

Pale stools and jaundice can also signal a very rare, potentially life-threatening liver disease, *biliary atresia*. This condition, which occurs in only 1 in 10,000 children, is usually first noted between the ages of 2 and 8 weeks. It's more common among full-term babies than preemies and is also more prevalent in girls than in boys. The highest incidence is in babies of Asian (especially Chinese) and African descent. The cause is unknown, but some believe that a virus or other infectious agent may be to blame.

In biliary atresia, the pale stools are usually noticed by the parents during the baby's first few weeks of life. Early diagnosis of biliary atresia is critical.

SIGN OF THE TIMES

Because of the importance of detecting biliary atresia in newborns, stool color charts are given to new parents in the United Kingdom, Japan, and some other countries to help them screen their infants for this and other potentially serious liver disorders.

Without immediate surgical treatment, it can lead to permanent liver damage (*cirrhosis*), liver failure, and death. If treatment is delayed beyond 3 months of age, the chance of survival beyond 2 years is very poor. However, when surgery is performed before the infant is 2 months old, a good outcome is much more likely. Unfortunately, even when surgery is successful, most babies will suffer some liver damage and may require special diets or other medical care. And they may eventually need a liver transplant.

Pale stools and jaundice can also signal hepatitis, an inflammation of the liver that can range from mild to serious. Most infants with hepatitis have relatively minor cases, with few if any associated signs. In severe cases, though, the baby may have fever, loss of appetite, fatigue, intense itching, abdominal pains, and vomiting as the disease progresses. These problems can usually be managed medically and further complications may be prevented with medication and special diets.

Last, acholic stools can also be a warning sign of cystic fibrosis (CF), a rare, inherited disease that causes serious respiratory and gastrointestinal problems. The stools may also be greasy and float (see **Floating Feces,** below), and the baby's skin may taste salty (see Chapter 8). Although there's no cure for CF, improved treatments have greatly increased the life expectancy of children with this disease.

WARNING SIGN

While most newborns are routinely screened for cystic fibrosis, not all states mandate such screening. Babies born in some foreign countries also may not have been screened for CF. If you're not certain if your baby was screened, mention it to his or her pediatrician.

BLACKISH POOP

Q: *Our 18-month-old son's stools have been very dark, almost black. What can cause this?*

A: Black stools can be a totally benign sign that a baby has been taking iron supplements, charcoal tablets (to control gas), or Pepto-Bismol or other stomach medicines containing bismuth. Eating a lot of black licorice, blueberries, and even some leafy green vegetables can also turn poop black.

If, however, the black stools are

SIGN OF THE TIMES

Recent research in the United Kingdom has uncovered the following about diaper changing:

- Only 1% of men change their babies' diapers.
- Those men who do change diapers do it faster than women (1 minute 36 seconds versus 2 minutes 5 seconds).

According to the researchers, men treat diaper changing like a pit stop—they want to get it over with as quickly as possible. The worse the smell, the quicker the change.

tarry and smelly too—medically known as *melena*—their color and consistency may be the result of bleeding in the upper gastrointestinal (GI) tract. Melena may signal *gastritis* (an inflammation of the stomach lining), which can be caused by bacterial or viral infections as well as by certain medications, including ibuprofen and other nonsteroidal anti-inflammatory drugs (NSAIDs). Persistent melena can be a warning sign of stomach ulcers or, in rare cases, tumors in the upper GI tract. Treatment depends on the cause of the bleeding.

REDDISH POOP

Q: Our toddler sometimes has bowel movements that look more red than brown. Could there be blood in them?

A: Not necessarily. Reddish stools may merely be a benign sign that your baby has been eating or drinking large amounts of red-colored food or beverages. Beets, tomato juice, red gelatin, red fruit punches, red ice pops, and red-colored liquid medicines are all common culprits.

That said, red or maroon stools may indeed contain blood. Bright red specks or streaks that are spotted on a baby's stools, diaper, or baby wipes or in his or her potty may be blood. Medically known as *hematochezia,* blood in stools is usually a sign of bleeding from the lower GI tract and can signal a variety of problems from minor to serious. The most common causes are milk allergies and constipation (hard stools can damage delicate tissue, causing bleeding). Some antibiotics and other medications can cause hematochezia. In these less serious cases, the bleeding will usually stop when the irritant is taken away. For example, if the bleeding is caused by a milk allergy, it will likely stop if the baby stops ingesting milk.

WARNING SIGN

Hematochezia can be caused by the insertion of sharp objects into the rectum by the baby or even someone else. In fact, in rare cases, blood in the stools can be an important warning sign of sexual abuse.

Red-currant-jelly-like stools in a baby who is crying, seems to be in a lot of pain, and has a fever and/or is vomiting can be a sign of *intussusception*. This is a rare bowel disorder in which one part of the intestine telescopes into another, cutting off the blood supply. This is the most common abdominal emergency in children under the age of 2. If it's not treated within 24 hours, the baby may go into shock, suffer from irreversible tissue damage, and even die.

Reddish or maroon stools may also signal a variety of intestinal infections and even parasites. In these cases, other signs such as diarrhea, nausea, and pain will likely be present. Depending on the cause, treatment may involve antibiotics or other medication.

In rare cases, persistently passing reddish or maroon stools in toddlers can be a warning sign of *ulcerative colitis* or *Crohn's disease*, which go under the umbrella term *inflammatory bowel disease* (IBD). These are chronic, potentially debilitating gastrointestinal disorders that tend to run in families.

Babies with IBD are likely to have other disturbing GI signs including diarrhea, cramps, nausea and vomiting, and weight loss. Depending on the severity, treatment might involve special diets, anti-inflammatory drugs including steroids, antibiotics, and occasionally surgery.

OTHER POOP PROBLEMS

WATERY STOOLS

Q: Our newly adopted baby girl has recently started having watery bowel movements several times a day. She doesn't seem to be sick. Is this normal or does she have diarrhea?

A: Your daughter's loose stools may be normal or diarrhea, depending on

SIGNS OF THE TIMES

Recent stool studies in Holland, the United Kingdom, and Turkey have discovered that:

- Breast-fed babies have more frequent bowel movements but produce smaller amounts of stool than bottle-fed babies.
- Most babies poop 3 to 6 times a day during the 1st month of life, and once a day from the 2nd to the 24th month.

her age. Some newborns will have many very watery, yellow bowel movements (up to 10 a day). Medically referred to as *transitional diarrhea,* this is perfectly normal and can last for up to 2 weeks.

Diarrhea is often defined as having loose, watery stools more than 3 times in one day. The stools may contain pus, mucus, and/or blood (see **Reddish Poop,** above). Most of the time, diarrhea is related to an infectious illness. In babies, diarrhea can be a sign of a food allergy, so if a baby develops diarrhea after he or she is first introduced to a new food, then that food might be the culprit.

Diarrhea can also be a reaction to antibiotics and other medications. But if a baby is bloated, seems in pain, vomits, and/or has a fever, the diarrhea may be a warning sign of a bacterial or viral infection or parasites.

WARNING SIGN

A recent study in Germany found that babies who are taken into chlorinated public pools during the first year of life are at increased risk for diarrhea. The researchers believe that this is because babies have immature lungs and immune systems, making them vulnerable to pool pollutants.

Chronic diarrhea, especially with weight loss, can occasionally be a telltale sign of one of several *malabsorption disorders,* conditions in which the body can't properly digest or efficiently absorb nutrients from the intestinal tract. Other signs may include bloating, gas, and abdominal pain. Celiac disease (see **Recurrent Runs,** below), *lactose intolerance* (see **Gassy Baby,** below), and IBD (see **Reddish Poop,** above)

WARNING SIGNS

Prolonged or severe diarrhea can cause dehydration, which can be life-threatening in babies.

Here are signs of dehydration in babies:

- A dry mouth and tongue
- Crying without tears
- No wet diapers for 3 hours or more
- A high fever
- Unusual sleepiness or drowsiness
- Sunken eyes

are among the most common of these disorders in older babies. If left untreated, malabsorption disorders can cause anemia, delayed growth, weight loss, malnutrition, and various life-threatening conditions.

Many medicines are available to stop diarrhea and prevent dehydration. However, in severe or chronic cases, the underlying cause for the diarrhea will need to be found and treated.

RECURRENT RUNS

Q: *Our toddler has been having bouts of diarrhea on and off for the past few months. He's also eating a variety of solids. My mother thinks he may have a wheat allergy. Would this cause diarrhea?*

A: Your mother is probably referring to celiac disease, one of the most common malabsorption disorders. (See **Watery Stools,** above.) Also known as *sprue,* it can indeed cause repeated bouts of diarrhea. Celiac disease is an inherited autoimmune disorder that usually makes its first appearance in older babies (it rarely manifests itself in infants). It's characterized by intolerance to gluten, a protein found in wheat, barley, rye, and—to a lesser extent—oats. When someone with sprue eats these grains, the gluten damages the lining of their small intestine. Corn and rice don't contain gluten and are therefore safe for babies with celiac disease.

Other common signs of celiac disease include floating, foul-smelling

SIGNS OF THE TIMES

- Celiac disease was first described in the 1st century A.D. by the ancient Greek physician Aretaeus.
- The word *gluten,* which comes from the Latin word for "glue," was first used in the 19th century to describe the sticky stuff that helps form dough.
- Because of its stickiness, gluten has long been used to make glue and, since the 1950s, Play-Doh.

WARNING SIGN

If your baby has celiac disease, carefully read all of the labels on his or her medications, foods, and beverages, since they may contain wheat, rye, or barley. And keep him or her away from stickers, stamps, envelopes, and anything else that has glue on it. Glue often contains gluten, and even a single lick can cause a severe reaction.

If a baby has been defini-
tively diagnosed with celiac
disease, the following 6 elements
are essential for treatment:

C—Consultation with a skilled
dietitian

E—Education about the disease

L—Lifelong adherence to a
gluten-free diet

I—Identification and treatment of
nutritional deficiencies

A—Access to an advocacy group

C—Continuous long-term
follow-up

stools, bloating, gas (see **Floating Feces** and **Gassy Baby,** below), pain, irritability, and failure to grow or gain weight. Interestingly, celiac disease can also cause constipation. It affects girls more often than boys and is more common among whites of European— especially Irish—ancestry. It's also more prevalent in families with a history of other autoimmune diseases.

Unfortunately, some parents mistak- enly assume their baby has celiac dis- ease, unnecessarily restricting his or her diet. Celiac disease needs to be carefully diagnosed. While there are blood tests that can be used to screen for this disease, to make a definitive diagnosis an intestinal biopsy—a very simple procedure—should be done by a gastroenterologist. Treatment in- volves being on a totally gluten-free diet for life. Nutritional supplements and certain medications, such as corticosteroids, may also be recommended.

PERIODIC POOPING

Q: My 2-year-old grandson usually goes several days without a bowel movement. I'm worried he's constipated, but his mother says this is perfectly normal and nothing to be concerned about. Who's right?

A: You both may be correct. When a baby has difficulty passing stools and/or the stools are hard and dry, he or she is most likely constipated. But if a baby poops without straining and his or her stools are soft, there's probably nothing to be concerned about.

While many babies have bowel movements every day, others do so only once every 3 or 4 days. Some medical definitions of constipation are (1) not having a bowel movement in 5 days, (2) having fewer than 3 bowel movements in a week, or (3) difficulty in passing small, hard, dry stools for 2 or more weeks.

Constipation has a variety of causes, from diet to disease. For exam- ple, while exclusively breast-fed babies are rarely constipated, formula-

Besides very infrequent bowel movements, other signs of constipation include:
- Hard, pebble-sized poop
- Grunting during bowel movements
- A streak of blood in the stool

fed babies may become constipated as a reaction to one of the ingredients in the formula. Constipation is also common when a baby is weaned from the breast or bottle and starts eating solid foods. The first solids a baby eats, such as rice, are often low in fiber. Fiber is necessary to add bulk to the stool and help it retain water, making it easier to pass. A fiber-rich diet will often help relieve constipation, but a doctor may also recommend a laxative or other medicine.

SIGNIFICANT FACT

A normal stool is about 75% water. If a baby's stool contains too little water, it becomes hard and often small and pebbly, and the baby becomes constipated. If the stools contain too much water, they'll be too soft. The end result— diarrhea.

Constipation can also be a warning sign that a baby is, or is becoming, dehydrated from not drinking enough fluid or from a fever or diarrhea. Alternatively, it may signal a medical problem such as *hypothyroidism,* an underactive thyroid. Other signs of hypothyroidism in babies

SIGNIFICANT FACT

The word *bowel* is derived from the Latin word for "sausage."

may include a slow heartbeat (*bradycardia*), large soft spots on the skull (see Chapter 1), poor growth, intolerance to cold, and hair loss (see Chapter 2). Treating the thyroid problem usually helps relieve the constipation. Other, less common causes of chronic constipation include celiac disease (see **Recurrent Runs,** above), cystic fibrosis (see Chapter 8 and **Pale Poop,** above), and diabetes (see **Peeing a Lot,** above).

In very rare cases (1 in 10,000 children), constipation can be a sign of *Hirschsprung's disease*, a congenital, potentially life-threatening blockage of the colon. Although Hirschsprung's disease can sometimes be so mild that it goes undiagnosed until adolescence or later, it's usually caught in infancy, when the newborn doesn't pass meconium within 48 hours of birth. (See **Yellowish Poop,** above.) Other signs of this disease in babies include pencil-thin stools, a swollen abdomen, slow growth and development, vomiting bile, and explosive diarrhea.

The cause of Hirschsprung's is unknown, but it occasionally runs in families. It's 5 times more prevalent in boys than in girls, and much more common in babies with Down syndrome and other genetic disorders.

Surgery is the only treatment for Hirschsprung's. When performed early, it can restore bowel function to normal in most babies. Delay in diagnosis and treatment decreases a baby's chances of ever having a functioning bowel.

FLOATING FECES

Q: *When our 2½-year-old son uses a toilet, I've noticed that his stools frequently float. I've heard that this can be a bad sign. Is that true?*

A: Most stools sink to the bottom of the toilet bowl. It's usually excess gas, from fiber-rich or other gas-producing foods, that keeps them afloat. (See **Gassy Baby,** below.) If the gas that causes the "floaters" is the by-product of a gastrointestinal infection, the baby will also likely have diarrhea. When the infection clears up, his or her stools will once again sink.

Frequent "floaters" can signal malabsorption disorders, including celiac disease (see **Recurrent Runs,** above), cystic fibrosis (see Chapter 8 and **Pale Poop,** above), or IBD (see **Reddish Poop** and **Watery Stools,** above). In general, babies with these problems will also have diarrhea and foul-smelling feces.

Floating, frothy, foul-smelling feces that have an oily coating (medically known as *steatorrhea*) are signs of an abnormally high amount of fat in the stool. They may be a telltale indication that the baby's diet is too rich in fat, but they could also be an important warning sign of malabsorption disorders and IBD. (See **Watery Stools** and **Reddish Poop,** above). In addition, steatorrhea may be the result of a blocked bile duct and may signal a liver disease. (See **Pale Poop,** above.)

GASSY BABY

Q: *Our baby passes a lot of gas. Can he be allergic to milk or have something else wrong with him?*

A: It's normal for babies to pass gas through the anus (a fart) or mouth (a burp). In some cases when a young baby has excessive gas, it can, indeed, signal a *cow's milk allergy* (CMA). Other signs may include diarrhea, fussiness, a skin rash, and wheezing.

CMA, which is an adverse reaction of the child's immune system to the protein in milk, is the most common food allergy of early childhood. It affects up to 5% of infants between the ages of 1 and 3 months, and typically resolves by 12 months of age.

Cow's milk allergy is sometimes confused with *lactose intolerance* (LI). But while CMA is an immunological condition that can also affect the skin and respiratory system, LI is strictly a gastrointestinal problem; a person with LI can't digest lactose, a sugar found in all milk products. And CMA primarily affects babies, while LI rarely affects children under the age of 4. (However, in African American children, lactose intolerance often occurs as early as age 2.)

Excessive gas emissions in older babies and toddlers may also be the

SIGN OF THE TIMES

Although the medical term *flatulence* is used to describe intestinal gas, there's no single medical term for the act of passing or expelling gas. The word *fart,* which has been popular since Chaucer's day, has become so widely accepted that the section on flatulence in the encyclopedic *Oxford Companion to the Body* is simply titled "Farting."

SIGNIFICANT FACTS

Lactose intolerance is extremely common in older children and adults of Asian, African, Ashkenazi Jewish, and Native American descent. It affects up to 80% of these populations.

SIGNIFICANT FACT

According to Nebraska law,
if a child burps in church,
the parents can be arrested! This ar-
chaic law is reported to still be on
the books.

result of eating high-fiber and other gas-producing foods, such as dried fruits. Or it may be a sign of celiac disease (see **Recurrent Runs,** above).

Frequent farting in a baby who has alternating bouts of diarrhea and constipation may signal *irritable bowel syndrome* (*IBS*), a common disorder of the intestines that leads to cramping, bloating, and changes in bowel habits. IBS (aka *spastic colon*) is considered a "functional" disease; that is, it causes discomfort and distress but is not associated with any other serious signs or diseases. The cause is unknown, but researchers believe that children and adults with IBS are more sensitive to gas or stool in the colon. IBS treatment usually involves dietary changes and medications to control the diarrhea, constipation, and cramping.

IBS shouldn't be confused with *IBD* (*inflammatory bowel disease*), a term that encompasses Crohn's disease and ulcerative colitis. Although children with IBD also may have excessive gas, they usually suffer from much more serious intestinal problems. (See **Reddish Poop,** above.)

Once the underlying cause of the excessive gas is diagnosed and treated, the problem should pass. In the meantime, some doctors may also recommend certain medications as a stopgap measure.

SIGNING OFF

The American Academy of Pediatrics recommends that babies born in hospitals or birthing centers not go home until they urinate. And if the baby doesn't pass meconium—the blackish, sticky substance that is the baby's first bowel movement—during his or her hospital stay, the parents will be told to be on the lookout for it at home. Once home, it's up to the parents to notice any unusual urinary or bowel-related signs and mention them to the baby's doctor. Some of these signs may be benign, but some may require immediate attention.

NOTIFY YOUR CHILD'S HEALTHCARE PROVIDER AS SOON AS POSSIBLE IF YOUR BABY:
- Has been having fewer wet diapers than usual
- Has been having much wetter diapers than usual and is exceedingly thirsty
- Has bloody urine
- Appears to be in pain when urinating or defecating
- Has had a recent and persistent change in bowel habits or stools
- Has what looks like spots or streaks of blood in the diaper or stool

NOTIFY YOUR CHILD'S HEALTHCARE PROVIDER IMMEDIATELY OR GO TO THE EMERGENCY ROOM IF YOUR BABY:
- Is constipated, vomiting, and seems to be in pain
- Has bloody diarrhea
- Has severe diarrhea and shows signs of dehydration

A general pediatrician can diagnose and treat most urinary and gastrointestinal conditions found in babies. But some disorders may require evaluation and treatment by a pediatric specialist. A child may therefore be referred to a urologist, gastroenterologist, nephrologist, or pediatric surgeon, among others. Sometimes parents of infants and babies with certain medical problems will also be referred to a geneticist, ethicist, and/or psychotherapist.

APPENDIX I

MULTISYSTEM DISEASES IN BABIES AND THEIR SIGNS

MANY POTENTIALLY SERIOUS DISEASES in babies can affect several different and seemingly unrelated body parts and systems. Because of this, many of these disorders are often under- or misdiagnosed or—at the very least—their diagnosis is delayed. With babies, especially, early diagnosis and treatment can be critical.

The following are some of the more common multisystem diseases that affect babies, and their most common signs. Babies with these conditions may have only a few of these signs or may have many of them. If you're at all concerned that your child may have one of these disorders, discuss it with his or her pediatrician as soon as possible.

CHILDHOOD CANCER

Cancers in infants and babies are extremely rare. The most common, *neuroblastoma,* occurs in only 65 out of 1 million babies. (Neuroblastoma is a malignant tumor that occurs most often in an infant's abdomen.) *Leukemia* (cancer of the white blood cells) is the second most common cancer, followed by *cancer of the central nervous system, retinoblastoma* (an eye cancer), and *Wilms' tumor* (a kidney cancer).

Childhood cancers are usually diagnosed before a baby is 2 years of age, most of the time by the baby's 1st birthday. Early diagnosis is essential to maximize the chances of successful treatment. The acronym CHILD CANCER below spells out the important warning signs of childhood cancer:

- Continued, unexplained weight loss
- Headaches, often with early-morning vomiting
- Increased swelling or persistent pain in bones, joints, back, or legs
- Lump(s) or mass(es), especially in the abdomen, neck, chest, pelvis, or armpits
- Development of excessive bruising, bleeding, or rashes
- Constant infections
- A "white reflex" in one eye in a photograph
- Nausea that persists, or vomiting without nausea
- Constant tiredness or noticeable paleness
- Eye or vision changes that occur suddenly and persist
- Recurrent or persistent fevers of unknown origin

CYSTIC FIBROSIS

Cystic fibrosis (*CF*) is a rare, inherited disease that causes serious respiratory and gastrointestinal problems in children. CF mostly affects white babies (1 in 3,000) and is extremely rare among other groups. Although there's no cure for CF, improved treatments have greatly increased the life expectancy of children with this disease.

Signs of cystic fibrosis in babies include:

- Very salty-tasting skin
- Excessive phlegm
- Persistent coughing
- Frequent lung or respiratory infections
- Wheezing or shortness of breath
- Poor growth or weight gain in spite of a good appetite
- Frequent diarrhea

- Pale, greasy, bulky, floating, foul-smelling stools
- Clubbed fingers and toes
- Distended belly

TYPE 1 (JUVENILE) DIABETES

Diabetes is a disease in which the body does not produce or properly use insulin. Type 1 diabetes affects about 1 in 600 children and is increasing at a rate of 5% a year among preschool children.

Signs of diabetes in babies include:

- Excessive thirst
- Constant hunger
- Excessive urination
- Sudden weight loss for no reason
- Rapid, hard breathing
- Sudden vision changes
- Weakness
- Drowsiness or exhaustion
- Fruity odor of breath
- Sweet-smelling urine
- Frequent bouts of candida (yeast infection)

HYPOTHYROIDISM

Hypothyroidism (aka *underactive thyroid*) is a condition in which the thyroid gland produces inadequate amounts of thyroxin, the hormone responsible for metabolism. Hypothyroidism affects about 1 in 4,000 babies born in the United States. If it's not caught early, hypothyroidism can lead to growth retardation and mental disabilities as well as other serious medical problems. However, once this condition is diagnosed, the treatment for it is very effective.

Because of the many seemingly unrelated signs and symptoms, hypothyroidism is difficult to diagnose, especially in children under age 2.

Signs of hypothyroidism in babies include:

- Large or extra fontanelle (soft spot)
- Puffy face
- Swollen tongue
- Hoarse cry
- Thick, coarse hair that grows low on the forehead
- Hair loss
- Intolerance to cold
- Cold extremities
- Mottled skin
- Poor muscle tone
- Poor feeding
- Prolonged jaundice
- Umbilical hernia
- Slow heartbeat
- Excessive sleepiness, tires easily
- Persistent constipation
- Slow to no growth

APPENDIX II

RESOURCES

In writing this book, we used many different medical and scientific sources, including textbooks, journals, and websites sponsored by the National Institutes of Health and other professional organizations. In addition, we found many consumer-oriented websites and books extremely helpful. Below is a list that you might also find useful and interesting.

RECOMMENDED WEBSITES

American Academy of Allergy, Asthma & Immunology www.aaaai.org

American Academy of Audiology www.audiology.org

American Academy of Dermatology www.aad.org

American Academy of Family Physicians www.aafp.org

American Academy of Otolaryngic Allergy www.aaoaf.org

American Academy of Otolaryngology—Head and Neck Surgery www.entnet.org

American Academy of Pediatric Dentistry www.aapd.org

American Academy of Pediatrics www.aap.org

American Association for Klinefelter Syndrome Information and Support www.aaksis.org

American Association of Oral and Maxillofacial Surgeons www.aaoms.org

American Cancer Society www.cancer.org

American College of Allergy, Asthma & Immunology www.acaai.org

American College of Rheumatology www.rheumatology.org

American Dental Association www.ada.org

American Diabetes Association www.diabetes.org

American Hearing Research Foundation www.american-hearing.org

American Lung Association www.lungusa.org

American Sleep Apnea Association www.sleepapnea.org

American Society of Plastic Surgeons www.plasticsurgery.org

American Speech-Language-Hearing Association www.asha.org

Arthritis Foundation www.arthritis.org

Asthma and Allergy Foundation of America www.aafa.org

Autism Society www.autism-society.org

Celiac Disease Foundation www.celiac.org

Centers for Disease Control www.cdc.gov/DiseasesConditions/

Centers for Disease Control: Infants and Toddlers www.cdc.gov/LifeStages/infants_toddlers.html

Children's Brain Tumor Foundation http://cbtf.org/cms

Children's Eye Foundation www.childrenseyefoundation.org

Children's Tumor Foundation www.ctf.org

Congenital Adrenal Hyperplasia Research Education &
Support (CARES) www.caresfoundation.org

Crohn's & Colitis Foundation of America www.ccfa.org

CureSearch Children's Oncology Group, National Childhood
Cancer Foundation www.curesearch.org

Cystic Fibrosis Foundation www.cff.org

Dysautonomia Foundation www.familialdysautonomia.org

Ehlers-Danlos National Foundation www.ednf.org

Endocrine Society www.endo-society.org

HealthFinder: U.S. Dept. of Health and Human Services
www.healthfinder.gov

Hormone Foundation www.hormone.org

Hypospadias & Epispadias Association www.heainfo.org

Juvenile Diabetes Research Foundation www.jdrf.org

KidsHealth (Nemours Foundation) www.kidshealth.org

Leukemia & Lymphoma Society www.leukemia-lymphoma.org

MAGIC Foundation for Children's Growth
www.magicfoundation.org

Maple Syrup Urine Disease (MSUD) Family Support Group
www.msud-support.org

March of Dimes Birth Defects Foundation
www.marchofdimes.com

Mayo Clinic www.mayoclinic.com

Medline Plus, U.S. National Library of Medicine and the
National Institutes of Health www.nlm.nih.gov/medlineplus

Merck Manuals Online Medical Library
www.merck.com/mmhe/index.html

National Adrenal Diseases Foundation www.nadf.us

National Alopecia Areata Foundation www.naaf.org

National Cancer Institute www.cancer.gov

National Center for Immunization and Respiratory Diseases (Centers for Disease Control and Prevention) www.cdc.gov/vaccines

National Center for Zoonotic, Vector-Borne, and Enteric Diseases, Division of Parasitic Diseases (Centers for Disease Control and Prevention) www.cdc.gov/ncidod/dpd/

National Diabetes Information Clearinghouse (NIH-National Institute of Diabetes and Digestive and Kidney Diseases) www.diabetes.niddk.nih.gov

National Dissemination Center for Children with Disabilities www.nichcy.org

National Down Syndrome Society www.ndss.org

National Eye Institute www.nei.nih.gov

National Foundation for Ectodermal Dysplasias http://nfed.org

National Graves' Disease Foundation www.ngdf.org

National Heart, Lung, and Blood Institute www.nhlbi.nih.gov

National Institute of Allergy and Infectious Diseases www3.niaid.nih.gov

National Institute of Arthritis and Musculoskeletal and Skin Diseases www.niams.nih.gov

National Institute of Child Health and Human Development www.nichd.nih.gov

National Institute of Diabetes and Digestive and Kidney Diseases www2.niddk.nih.gov

National Institute of Environmental Health Sciences www.niehs.nih.gov

National Institute of Neurological Disorders and Stroke
www.ninds.nih.gov

National Institute on Deafness and Other Communication
Disorders www.nidcd.nih.gov

National Kidney and Urologic Diseases Information
Clearinghouse (National Institute of Diabetes and Digestive
and Kidney Diseases) www.kidney.niddk.nih.gov

National Kidney Foundation www.kidney.org

National Library of Medicine www.nlm.nih.gov

National Marfan Foundation www.marfan.org

National Network for Immunization Information
www.immunizationinfo.org

National Organization for Albinism and Hypopigmentation
www.albinism.org

National Organization for Rare Disorders www.rarediseases.org

National Scoliosis Foundation www.scoliosis.org

National Vaccine Program Office (United States Department
of Health and Human Services) www.hhs.gov/nvpo

National Vitiligo Foundation www.nvfi.org

Osteogenesis Imperfecta Foundation www.oif.org

Pediatric Brain Tumor Foundation www.pbtfus.org

Save Babies Through Screening Foundation www.savebabies.org

Spina Bifida Association www.sbaa.org

United Cerebral Palsy www.ucp.org

U.S. Food and Drug Administration www.fda.gov

U.S. National Library of Medicine www.ncbi.nlm.nih.gov/pubmed

Xeroderma Pigmentosum (XP) Society www.xps.org

BOOKS

Babies: History, Art, and Folklore
Beatrice Fontanel and Claire d'Harcourt
Harry N. Abrams, 1997

Childhood and Children: A Compendium of Customs, Superstitions, Theories, Profiles, and Facts
Joan Bel Geddes
Oryx Press, United States, 1997

Folk-lore from Adams County, Illinois
Harry Middleton Hyatt
Alma Egan Foundation, 1935
www.qucommunication.com/FACIpdf.pdf

The Oxford Companion to the Body
Edited by Colin Blakemore and Sheila Jennett
Oxford University Press, England, 2001

Small World: A History of Baby Care from the Stone Age to the Spock Age
Joan Bel Geddes
Macmillan, United States, 1964

Yesterday's Children: The Antiques and History of Childcare
Sally Kevill-Davies
Antique Collectors' Club, England, 1991

ACKNOWLEDGMENTS

We would like to thank our agent, Kris Dahl, who was there at the conception of both *Body Signs* and *Baby Body Signs* and had the foresight to put us into the capable and caring hands of Beth Rashbaum, senior editor at Bantam. We're very grateful to Beth for helping us through the gestation period, and to Angela Polidoro, who skillfully and painlessly guided us through the long labor and delivery of the book. We also thank the rest of the crew at Bantam, especially Margaret Benton, Christopher Zucker, and Belina Huey.

To the talented artist Nenad Jakesevic, who was responsible for the many wonderful illustrations that grace the pages of this book as well as our previous one, we extend our heartfelt gratitude.

A very special thanks to B. J. Carter for suggesting that Dr. Woodie Kessel write the foreword. And we are indebted to Dr. Kessel for agreeing to do so, and for his thoughtful and thought-provoking essay.

We're extremely grateful to each member of our panel of medical experts for selflessly sharing their time, expertise, advice, and editing skills: Dr. Keith J. Benkov, Dr. Wilma Bergfeld, Dr. Steven Grossman, Dr. Joseph Haddad, Dr. Brenda Kohn, Dr. Charles Merker, Dr. Walter J. Molofsky, Dr. Karen Onel, Dr. David R. Roth, Dr. Peter Smith, and Dr. Christine L. Williams.

Dr. Dalit Ashany, Dr. Jonathon Aviv, Dr. Loren Greene, Dr. Ronald Kraft, Dr. Sharon Lewin, and Dr. Shelley Peck provided helpful suggestions as well as encouragement, and Mary Diamond at the

Cleveland Clinic once again came through for us. We'd also like to acknowledge Karen Drucker Omahen, Deirdre Omahen, Vivian Lang, Dr. Nicole Lang Gems, and all the other parents and grandparents who contributed topics for our Q&As.

We thank Richard Liebmann-Smith not only for his incomparable editing skills, but for his patience in putting up with the "Joan and Jacquie Show" weekend after weekend. And a special thanks to Dr. John Stangel and Vicky Baldwin of the Center for Advanced Reproductive Services for introducing us to each other at IVF Australia, where we first collaborated.

Joan would also like to thank Orit Spanier, Sara Berg, Paula Atkinson and the rest of the staff at the JCC Manhattan, who helped keep her in good physical shape and spirits throughout the writing of this book. And she will be forever grateful to her daughter Rebecca's wonderful pediatricians—Dr. Ramon Murphy, Dr. Signe Larsen, and Dr. Beth Cohen—for their careful attention to Rebecca's baby body signs, and to Dr. Ronald Kraft and Dr. Laura Schiller for successfully weaning her away from her beloved pediatricians. And Jacqueline would like to acknowledge the superb care that Pediatric Associates in Rye Brook, New York, gave to her daughter Elizabeth during her growing years. Drs. Norman Berkowitz and Jeffrey L. Brown always knew that listening to a parent's concern is a vital step in caring for a child.

Finally, unbeknownst to him, Jonathan Schwartz's soothing voice and the marvelous music he played on his National Public Radio show helped sustain us through countless hours at our computers.

INDEX

Page numbers of illustrations appear in italics

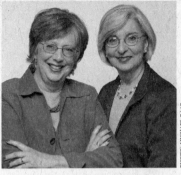

PHOTO: MICHAEL RAAB

Joan Liebmann-Smith (*left*)
Jacqueline Nardi Egan (*right*)

Joan Liebmann-Smith, Ph.D., is a medical writer and medical sociologist who specializes in health promotion and disease prevention in women and children. She was program manager of the American Health Foundation's child health promotion program, *Know Your Body,* and assistant director of the Maternity Center Association. Currently she is a consultant for Healthy Directions' Healthy Children Healthy Futures program.

Dr. Liebmann-Smith received her B.A. from New York University and her Ph.D. from the Graduate Center of the City University of New York. She is a past recipient of the American Medical Association's Medical Reporting Award. Her articles have appeared in many national magazines including *American Health, Ms., Newsweek, Redbook, Self,* and *Vogue,* as well as on various medical websites. She and her co-author, Jacqueline Nardi Egan, have written three previous books together: *Body Signs: From Warning Signs to False Alarms . . . How to Be Your Own Diagnostic Detective* (2007), *The Unofficial Guide to Getting Pregnant* (2005), and *The Unofficial Guide to Overcoming Infertility* (1999). Also the author of *In Pursuit of Pregnancy* (1989), Dr. Liebmann-Smith has appeared on such national television shows as *The Oprah Winfrey Show,* the *Today* show, and *The Early Show.*

Dr. Liebmann-Smith sits on the board of directors of the National Council on Women's Health. She holds memberships in the National Association of Science Writers, the American Medical Writers Association, and the American Sociological Association. She lives in New York City with her husband, Richard, also a writer. They have a twenty-six-year-old daughter, Rebecca, and a rescue cat, Fazelnut.

Jacqueline Nardi Egan is a medical journalist who specializes in developing and writing educational programs with and for physicians, allied health professionals, patients, and consumers. Currently she is director of editorial program development at QD Healthcare Group and Continuing Education Alliance in Stamford, Connecticut, and is a former medical editor of *Family Health* magazine. Ms. Egan has appeared on local and national radio and television shows, including *The Early Show* and *Weekend Today* in New York. She has a daughter, Elizabeth, and two rescue dogs, Coco and Abby; she divides her time between Darien, Connecticut, and Sag Harbor, New York.